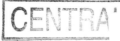

BESTMEDICINE

Atopic eczema

Dr George Kassianos
Dr Roger Allen
Dr Stephen Kownacki
Dr Tim Mitchell

Foreword by Claire Rayner
President of the Patients Association

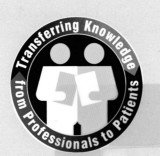

Managing Editor: Dr Scott Chambers
Medical Writers: Dr Eleanor Bull, Dr Anna Palmer, Dr Rebecca Fox-Spencer
Editorial Controller: Emma Catherall
Operations Manager: Julia Potterton
Designer: Chris Matthews
Typesetter: Julie Smith
Glossary: Dr Susan Chambers
Indexer: Laurence Errington
Director – Online Business: Peter Llewellyn
Publishing Director: Julian Grover
Publisher: Stephen I'Anson

© 2005 CSF Medical Communications Ltd.

1 Bankside
Lodge Road
Long Hanborough
Oxfordshire
OX29 8LJ, UK
Tel: +44 (0)1993 885370
Fax: +44 (0)1993 881868
Email: *enquiries@bestmedicine.com*

www.bestmedicine.com
www.csfmedical.com

The content of *BESTMEDICINE* is the work of a number of authors and has been produced in line with our standard editorial procedures, including the peer review of the disease overview and the drug reviews, and the passing of the final manuscript for publication by the Managing Editor and the Editor-in-Chief or the Medical Editor. Whilst every effort has been made to ensure the accuracy of the information at the date of approval for publication, the Authors, the Publisher, the Editors and the Editorial Board accept no responsibility whatsoever for any errors or omissions or for any consequences arising from anything included in or excluded from *BESTMEDICINE*.

All reasonable effort is made to avoid infringement of copyright law, including the redrawing of figures adapted from other sources. Where copyright permission has been deemed necessary, attempts are made to gain appropriate permission from the copyright holder. However, the Authors, the Publisher, the Editors and the Editorial Board accept no personal responsibility for any infringement of copyright law howsoever made. Any queries regarding copyright approvals or permissions should be addressed to the Managing Editor.

You are strongly urged to consult your doctor before taking, stopping or changing any of the products reviewed or referred to in *BESTMEDICINE* or any other medication that has been prescribed or recommended by your doctor.

A catalogue record for this book is available from the British Library.

ISBN: 1-905064-95-0

Typeset by Creative, Langbank, Scotland.
Printed and bound by KHL Printing Co PTE Ltd, Singapore.
Distributed by NBN International, Plymouth, Devon.

Contents

Foreword

Claire Rayner
President of The Patients Association

Patients and their families are rightly entitled to have access to good-quality, independent and reliable information concerning a diverse range of conditions and a wide variety of medications that are available to treat them. Indeed, there is a growing recognition amongst the majority of healthcare professionals that well-informed patients are more likely to adopt a more active role in the management of their illness and will therefore feel more satisfied with the care that they receive. Such an effect has the potential not only to directly benefit the patient and their families, but can also maximise limited healthcare resources within an already over-stretched NHS. However, at present access to this kind of information is limited, despite the fact that as many as one-in-four adults (12 million people in the UK alone) want ready access to this knowledge prior to visiting their doctor.

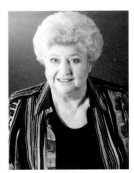

Photograph courtesy of
Amanda Rayner

The importance of patient self-management is a key component of current NHS strategy. Indeed, this has been widely acknowledged in an NHS-led campaign called the Expert Patient Programme (*www.expertpatient.nhs.uk*). This is a self-management course which aims to give people the confidence, skills and knowledge to manage their condition better and take greater control of their lives. The Expert Patient Programme defines an Expert Patient as one who has had the condition for long enough to have learnt the language doctors use.

BESTMEDICINE aims to meet the information and educational needs of both patients and healthcare professionals alike. The information found in the *BESTMEDICINE* series will assist patients and their families to obtain the level of information they now need to understand and manage their medical condition in partnership with their doctor. As *BESTMEDICINE* draws much of its content from medical publications written by doctors for doctors, some readers may find these books rather challenging when they first approach them. Despite this, I strongly believe that the effort that you invest in reading this book will be fully repaid by the increased knowledge that you will gain about this condition. Indeed, the extensive glossary of terms that can be found within each book certainly makes understanding the text a great deal easier, and the Patient Notes section is also very informative and reassuringly written by a doctor for the less scientifically minded reader. *BESTMEDICINE* represents the world's first source of independent, unabridged medical information that will appeal to patients and their families as well as healthcare professionals. This development should be welcomed and applauded, and I would commend these books to you.

Claire Rayner

Claire Rayner has been involved with the Patients Association for many years and has considerable expertise and experience from a professional background in nursing and journalism and her personal experience both as a patient and as a carer. She is well known as a leading 'Agony Aunt' and as a medical correspondent for many popular magazines. Claire has also published articles in a number of professional journals, as well as over forty medical, nursing and patient advice books.

An introduction to *BESTMEDICINE*

The source: information for healthcare professionals

Over the years, it has become increasingly apparent that there is a dearth of drug-related information that is independently compiled and robustly reviewed, and which also acknowledges the challenges faced by healthcare professionals when applying evidence-based medicine whilst practising at the 'front line' of patient care. As such, many healthcare professionals feel a certain ambivalence towards the numerous drug review publications that are currently on offer and, indeed, many do not have confidence in the information that can be found within their pages. In response to the need for a more impartial information resource – one that is independent of the pharmaceutical industry and the health service – we developed a novel publication, which was launched to meet this perceived lack of independent information. This peer-reviewed publication is called *Drugs in Context* and was launched in May 2003 and is the source of much of what you will find in this edition of *BESTMEDICINE*.

Uniquely independent

Drugs in Context is unique in that it reviews the significant clinical and pharmacological evidence underpinning the use of a single drug, in the disease area(s) where it is used and the practice setting where it is most commonly prescribed. Over 50 issues are published each year covering numerous diseases and conditions. The principal goal of *Drugs in Context* is to become the definitive drug and disease management resource for all healthcare professionals. As such, over the coming years, the publication plans to review all of the significant drugs that are currently used in clinical practice.

Reliable and impartial information for patients too

In addition to the lack of impartial information for the healthcare professional, we also firmly believe that there is a significant and growing number of patients who are not served well in this regard either. Indeed, it is becoming apparent to us that many patients would welcome access to the same sources of information on drugs and diseases that their doctors and other healthcare professionals have access to.

There are numerous sources of information currently available to patients – ranging from leaflets and books to websites and other electronic media. However, despite their best intentions, the rigour and accuracy of many of these resources cannot always be relied upon due to significant variation in the quality of the material. Perhaps the major problem facing a patient or a loved one who is hunting for specific information relating to a disease or the drug that has been prescribed by their doctor is that there is simply too much material available, making sifting through it to find a relevant fact akin to looking for a needle in a haystack! More importantly, many of these resources can often (albeit unintentionally) patronise the reader who has made every effort to actively seek out information that can serve to reassure themselves about the relevant illness and the medication(s) prescribed for it.

Can knowledge be the 'BESTMEDICINE'?

We firmly believe as healthcare professionals, that an informed patient is more likely to take an active role in the management of their disease or condition and, therefore, will be more likely to benefit from any course of treatment. This means that everyone will benefit – the patient, their family and friends, the healthcare professionals involved in their care, and the NHS and the country as a whole! Indeed, such is the importance of patient education, that the NHS has launched an initiative emphasising the need for patients to assume a more active role in the management of their condition via the acquisition of knowledge and skills related specifically to their disease. This initiative is called the Expert Patients Programme (*www.expertpatients.nhs.uk*).

Filling the need for quality information

Many of our observations about the lack of quality education have underpinned the principles behind the launch of *BESTMEDICINE*, much of the content of which is drawn directly from the pages of *Drugs in Context*, as written by and for healthcare professionals. *BESTMEDICINE* aims to appeal primarily to the patient, loved-one or carer who wants to improve their knowledge of the disease in question, the evidence for and against the drugs available to treat the disease and the practical challenges faced by healthcare professionals in managing it.

A whole new language!

We fully acknowledge that a lot of medical terminology used in order to expedite communication amongst the medical community will be new to many of you, some terms may be difficult to pronounce and sometimes surplus to requirements. However, rather than significantly abridge the content and risk excluding something of importance to the reader, we have instead provided you with a comprehensive glossary of terms and what we hope will be helpful additional GP discussion pieces at the end of each section to aid understanding further. We have also provided you with an introduction to the processes underlying drug development and the key concepts in disease management which we hope you will also find informative and which we strongly recommend that you read before tackling the rest of this edition of *BESTMEDICINE*.

No secrets

By providing the same information to patients and their families as healthcare professionals we believe that *BESTMEDICINE* will help to foster better relationships between patients, their families and doctors and other healthcare professionals, and ultimately may even improve treatment outcomes.

This edition is one of a number of unique collections of disease summaries and drug reviews that we will be making widely available over the coming months. You will find details about each issue as it is published at *www.bestmedicine.com*.

We do hope that you find this edition of *BESTMEDICINE* illuminating.

Dr George Kassianos, GP, Bracknell; Editor-in-Chief – *Drugs in Context*;
     Editor – *BESTMEDICINE*
Dr Jonathan Morrell, GP, Hastings; Medical Editor (Primary Care) –
     Drugs in Context
Dr Michael Schachter, Consultant Physician, St Mary's Hospital
     Paddington; Clinical Pharmacology Editor – *Drugs in Context*

Reader's guide

We acknowledge that some of the medical and scientific terminology used throughout *BESTMEDICINE* will be new to you and will address sometimes challenging concepts. However, rather than abridge the content and risk excluding important information, we have included this Reader's Guide to dissect and explain the contents of *BESTMEDICINE* in order to make it more digestible to the less scientifically minded reader. We recommend that you familiarise yourself with the drug development process, summarised below, before embarking on the Drug Reviews. This brief synopsis clarifies and contextualises many of the specialist terms encountered in the Drug Reviews.

Following this Reader's Guide, you will find that *BESTMEDICINE* is made up of three main sections – a Disease Overview, an overview of Management Options and individual Drug Reviews – all of which are evidence-based and as such have been highly referenced. All references are listed at the end of each section. Importantly, the manuscript has been 'peer-reviewed', which means that it has undergone rigorous checks for accuracy both by a practising doctor and a specialist in drug pharmacology. These sections are sandwiched between two opinion pieces, an Editorial, written by a recognised expert in the field, and an Improving Practice article, written by a practising GP with a specialist interest in the disease area. It is important to bear in mind that these authors are addressing their professional colleagues, rather than a 'lay' reader, providing you with a fascinating and unique insight into many of the challenges faced by doctors in the day-to-day practice of medicine.

The Disease Overview, Drug Reviews and Improving Practice sections are all followed by a short commentary by Dr Tim Mitchell entitled Patient Notes. In these sections, Dr Mitchell reiterates some of the key issues raised in rather more 'patient-friendly' language.

As mentioned previously, much of the content of *BESTMEDICINE* has been taken directly from *Drugs in Context*, which is written by and for healthcare professionals. Consequently, some of the language used may be difficult for the less scientifically minded reader. To help with this, in addition to the Patient Notes, we have included a comprehensive glossary of terms found throughout the text.

Disease overview

The disease overview provides a brief synopsis of the disease, its symptoms, diagnosis and a critique of the currently available treatment options.

- The epidemiology, or incidence and distribution of the disease within a population, is discussed, with particular emphasis on UK-specific data.
- The aetiology section describes the specific causes or origins of the disease, which are usually a result of both genetic and environmental

factors. Multifactorial diseases result from more than one causative element. If an individual has a genetic predisposition, they are more susceptible to developing the disease as a result of their genetic make-up.

● The functional changes that accompany a particular syndrome or disease constitute its pathophysiology.

● The management of a disease may be influenced by treatment guidelines, specific directives published by government agencies, professional societies, or by the convening of expert panels. The National Institute for Clinical Excellence (NICE), an independent sector of the NHS comprised of experts in the field of treatment, is one such body.

● The social and economic factors that characterise the influence of the disease, describe its socioeconomic impact. Such factors include the cost to the healthcare provider to treat the disease – in terms of GP consultations, drug costs and the subsequent burden on hospital resources – or the cost to the patient or employer with respect to the number of work days lost as a consequence of ill health.

This edition of *BESTMEDICINE* focuses on the topical calcineurin inhibitors and their use in atopic eczema. However, to give our readers further information regarding other available treatments for atopic eczema and other forms of eczema, we have also included an overview of other medications currently available (see Management Options – Atopic Eczema). Future editions of *BESTMEDICINE* will look at other drug treatment options.

Drug reviews

☞ *The pharmacokinetics of a drug are of interest to healthcare professionals because it is important for them to understand the action of a drug on the body over a period of time.*

The drug reviews are not intended to address every available treatment for a particular disease. Rather, we focus on the major drugs currently available in the UK for the treatment of the featured disease and evaluate their performance in clinical trials and their safety in clinical practice. The basic pharmacology of the drug – the branch of science that deals with the origin, nature, chemistry, effects and uses of drugs – is discussed initially. This includes a description of the mechanism of action of the drug, the manner in which it exerts its therapeutic effects, and its pharmacokinetics (or the activity of the drug within the body over a period of time). Pharmacokinetics encompasses the absorption of the drug into or across the tissues of the body, its distribution to specific functional areas, its metabolism – the process by which it is broken down within the body into by-products (metabolites) – and ultimately, its removal or excretion from the body. The most frequently used pharmacokinetic terms that are used in the drug review sections of *BESTMEDICINE* are explained in Table 1.

Table 1. Key pharmacokinetic terms.

Term	Definition
Agonist	A drug/substance that has affinity for specific cell receptors triggering a biological response.
Antagonist	A drug/substance that blocks the action of another by binding to a specific cell receptor without eliciting a biological response.
AUC (area under curve)	A plot of the concentration of a drug against the time since initial administration. It is a means of describing the bioavailability of a drug.
Binding affinity	An attractive force between substances that causes them to enter into and remain in chemical contact.
Bioavailability	The degree and rate at which a drug is absorbed into a living system or is made available at the site of physiological activity.
Clearance	The rate at which the drug is removed from the blood by excretion into the urine through the kidneys.
C_{max}	The maximum concentration of the drug recorded in the blood plasma.
Cytochrome P450 (CYP) system	A group of enzymes responsible for the metabolism of a number of different drugs and substances within the body.
Dose dependency	In which the effect of the drug is proportional to the concentration of drug administered.
Enzyme	A protein produced in the body that catalyses chemical reactions without itself being destroyed or altered. The suffix 'ase' is used when designating an enzyme.
Excretion	The elimination of a waste product (in faeces or urine) from the body.
Half-life ($t_{1/2}$)	The time required for half the original amount of a drug to be eliminated from the body by natural processes.
Inhibitor	A substance that reduces the activity of another substance.
Ligand	Any substance that binds to another and brings about a biological response.
Potency	A measure of the power of a drug to produce the desired effects.
Protein binding	The extent to which a drug attaches to proteins, peptides or enzymes within the body.
Receptor	A molecular structure, usually (but not always) situated on the cell membrane, which mediates the biological response that is associated with a particular drug/substance.
Synergism	A phenomenon in which the combined effects of two drugs are more powerful than when either drug is administered alone.
t_{max}	The time taken to reach the maximum concentration of drug in plasma.
Volume of distribution (V_D)	The total amount of drug in the body divided by its concentration in the blood plasma. Used as a measure of the dispersal of the drug within the body once it has been absorbed.

Whilst the basic pharmacology of a drug is clearly important, the main focus of each drug review is to summarise the drug's performance in controlled clinical trials. Clinical trials examine the effectiveness, or clinical efficacy, of the drug against the disease or condition it is licensed to treat, as well as its safety and tolerability – the side-effects associated with the drug and the likelihood that the patient will tolerate treatment. Adherence to drug treatment, or patient compliance, reflects the tendency of patients to comply with the terms of their treatment regimen. Compliance may be affected by treatment-related side-effects or the convenience of drug treatment. The safety of the drug also encompasses its contraindications – conditions under which the drug should never be prescribed. This may mean avoiding use in special patient populations (e.g. young or elderly patients, or those with co-existing or comorbid conditions, such as liver or kidney disease) or avoiding coadministration with certain other medications.

A brief synopsis of the drug development process is outlined below, in order to clarify and put into context many of the specialist terms encountered throughout the drug reviews.

The drug development process

Launching a new drug is an extremely costly and time-consuming venture. The entire process can cost an estimated £500 million and can take between 10 and 15 years from the initial identification of a potentially useful therapeutic compound in the laboratory to launching the finished product as a treatment for a particular disease (Figure 1). Much of this time is spent fulfilling strict guidelines set out by regulatory authorities, in order to ensure the safety and quality of the end product.

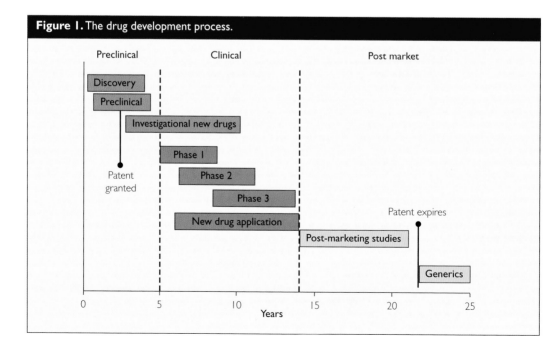

Figure 1. The drug development process.

As a consequence of this, a drug can fail at any stage of the development process and its development abandoned. Once identified and registered, the new drug can be protected by a patent for 20 years, after which time other companies are free to manufacture and market identical drugs, called generics. Thus, the pharmaceutical company has a finite period of time before patent expiry to recoup the cost of drug development (of both successful drugs and those drugs that do not make it to the marketplace) and return a profit to their shareholders.

Potential new drugs are identified by the research and development (R&D) department of the pharmaceutical company. After a candidate drug has been selected for development, it enters a rigorous testing procedure with five distinct phases – preclinical, which takes place in the laboratory, and phases 1, 2, 3 and 4, which involve testing in humans (Figure 1). Approval from the regulatory body is essential before the drug can be marketed and is dependent on the satisfactory completion of all phases of testing. In the UK, the Medicines and Healthcare products Regulatory Agency (MHRA) and the European Medicines Agency (EMEA) regulate the development process and companies must apply to these organisations for marketing authorisation. Within Europe, the Mutual Recognition Procedure means that the approval of a drug in one country (the Reference Member State), forms the basis for its subsequent approval in other European Union member states. This can make the approval process more efficient and may lead to approval being granted in several European countries at once. Once approval has been granted, the drug will be given a licence detailing the specific disease or conditions it is indicated to treat and the patient groups it may be used in. The drug will be assigned either prescription-only medicine (POM) or over-the-counter (OTC) status. POMs can only be obtained following consultation with a doctor, who will actively supervise their use.

Preclinical testing

Preclinical testing is essential before a drug can progress to human clinical trials. It is estimated that only one of every 1000 compounds that enter the preclinical stage continue into human testing (phases 1–4). Preclinical testing, or screening, is for the main-part performed in animals, and every effort is made to use as few animals as possible and to ensure their humane and proper care. Generally, two or more species (one rodent, one non-rodent) are tested, since a drug may affect one species differently from another.

Although a drug will never act in exactly the same way in animals as in humans, animal models are designed to mimic a human disease condition as closely as possible and provide information essential to drug development. *In vitro* experiments – literally meaning 'in glass' – are performed outside the living system in a laboratory setting. *In vivo* experiments are performed in the living cell or organism.

It is during the preclinical phase that the pharmacodynamics of the drug will first be examined. These include its mechanism of action, or the way in which it exerts its therapeutic effects. The drug's pharmacokinetics, toxicology (potentially hazardous or poisonous effects) and the formulation of the drug – the manner in which it is taken (e.g. tablet, injection, liquid) – are also assessed at this point in development.

Phase 1

Phase 1 trials are usually conducted in a small group of 10–80 healthy volunteers and further evaluate the biochemical and physiological effects of the drug – its chemical and biological impact within the body. An appropriate dosage range will be established at this point – the maximum and minimum therapeutic concentrations of the drug which are associated with a tolerable number of side-effects (secondary and usually adverse events unrelated to the beneficial effects of the drug). The mechanism of action and pharmacokinetic effects of the drugs are also further explored in this, the first group of human subjects to receive the drug.

Phase 2

If no major problems are revealed during phase 1 development, the drug can progress to phase 2 trials which take place in 100–300 patients diagnosed with the disease or condition that the drug is designed to treat. At this stage it is important to determine the effectiveness, or efficacy, of the drug. If the drug is no better than placebo then it will not be granted a licence. The side-effect or adverse event profile of the drug is re-examined at this stage, and is particularly pertinent in these patients, who may react more severely to the drug than healthy volunteers. The likelihood and severity of drug interactions is also of great importance in this patient group. Drug interactions – in which the action of one drug interferes with the action of another – can occur if the patient is taking more than one form of medication for the treatment of a comorbid disease or condition. If multiple drugs are administered together, or concomitantly, then the risk of drug interactions is increased.

Phase 3

Phase 3 clinical trials involve between 1000 and 3000 patients diagnosed with the relevant disease or condition. The recruitment of patients and the co-ordination and analysis of the trials is costly, so the pharmaceutical company will not embark on this stage unless they are sufficiently convinced of the therapeutic benefits of their drug. Essentially, phase 3 trials are replications of phase 2 trials but on a larger scale. The duration of the trial depends on the type of drug and the length of time required in order to determine the efficacy of the drug. For example, an antibiotic trial will have a shorter duration than a trial of a drug intended to treat long-term conditions, such as Alzheimer's disease. Acute treatment describes a short-term schedule given over a period of days or weeks, and chronic treatment refers to longer-term treatment schedules, lasting over periods of months or years.

Clinical trials may compare the new drug with an existing drug – a comparative trial – or may simply compare the new drug with no active drug treatment at all – a placebo-controlled trial. The participants who receive a comparator treatment or placebo are termed controls. In placebo-controlled trials, patients are given a placebo – an inert substance with no specific pharmacological activity – in place of the active drug. Patients will be unaware that the substance they are taking is placebo, which will be visually identical to the active treatment. This approach rules out any psychological effects of drug treatment – a patient may perceive that their condition has improved simply through the action of taking a tablet. In order to be considered clinically effective, the experimental drug must produce better results than the placebo.

The clinical trial should be designed in such a way as to limit the degree of bias it carries. The blinding of the trial is one means of eliminating bias. Double-blind trials, in which neither the doctor nor the patient knows which is the real drug and which is the placebo or comparator drug, are the most informative. In single-blind trials, only the patient is unaware of what they are taking, and in open-label trials, all participants are aware of treatment allocation. Conducting the trial across a number of clinics or hospitals, either abroad or in the same country (multicentre trials), further eliminates bias, as does randomisation, the random allocation of patients to treatment groups. At the start of the study, the baseline characteristics of the study population are recorded and are used as a starting point for all subsequent comparisons.

Efficacy is commonly measured by means of primary and secondary endpoints. Endpoints mark a recognised stage in the disease process and are used to compare the outcome in different treatment arms of clinical trials. The endpoint of one trial may be a marker of improvement or recovery whereas another trial may use the deterioration of the patient (morbidity) or death (mortality) to signify the end of the trial. Either way, endpoints represent valid criteria by which to compare treatments. On a similar note, surrogate markers are laboratory measurements of biological activity within the body that provide an indirect measure of the effect of treatment on disease state (e.g. blood pressure and cholesterol levels).

Statistical analysis allows the investigator to draw rational conclusions from clinical trials regarding the effectiveness of their drug. If the patient data generated during the course of a clinical trial are statistically significant, then there is a high probability that the given result, be it an improvement or a decline in the health of the patient, is due to a specific effect of drug treatment, rather than a chance occurrence. The data are put through a number of mathematical procedures that ultimately produce a p-value. This value reflects the probability that the result occurred by chance. For example, if the p-value is less than or equal to 0.05, the result is usually considered to be statistically significant. Such a p-value indicates that there is a 95% probability that the result did not occur by chance. The smaller the p-value, the more significant the result. When quoting clinical findings,

☛ Someone is always aware of who is taking what in a clinical trial. Whilst neither a doctor nor a patient may be aware of their treatment in a double-blind trial, there is a secure coding system, known only to the investigator, which contains the various treatment allocations.

the *p*-value is often given in brackets in order to emphasise the importance of the finding.

Once a drug has progressed through the key stages of development and demonstrated clear efficacy with an acceptable safety profile, the data are collated and the pharmaceutical company will then submit a licence application to the regulatory authorities – a new drug application.

Phase 4 (Post-marketing studies)

Phase 4 testing takes place after the drug has been marketed and involves large numbers of patients, sometimes including those groups that may have previously been excluded from clinical trials (e.g. pregnant women and elderly or young patients). These trials are usually open-label, so the patient is aware of what they are taking, without control groups. They provide valuable information regarding the tolerability of the drug, and may reveal any long-term adverse events associated with treatment. Post-marketing surveillance continues throughout the life-span of the drug, and constantly monitors its safety, usage and performance. Doctors are advised to inform the MHRA and the Committee on Safety of Medicines (CSM) of any adverse events they encounter. Patients can also alert the CSM of any adverse events they may experience through their website (*www.yellowcard.gov.uk*).

Editorial

Dr Roger Allen
Consultant Dermatologist, University Hospital
Queen's Medical Centre, Nottingham

Eczema, asthma, hay fever and allergies in general, are so much a part of the modern world that it is pertinent to remember that it was just over a century ago that atopy was first recognised as a clinical entity in its own right. An association between eczema, hay fever and asthma was first noted by Besnier in 1892 and the term 'atopy' itself was introduced by Coca and Cooke in 1923 to explain their belief that such symptoms arose from an inappropriate response to environmental factors. Since then the prevalence of atopy has risen relentlessly so that by the age of 7 years, 15% of children in the developed world can expect to have had at least one episode of eczema.

What has caused this rapid rise? Genetic factors certainly contribute but are unlikely to change at such a rate sufficient to be responsible for such a radical increase in prevalence. Therefore, our attention inevitably turns to environmental factors – but which ones? Are we guilty of polluting our world with toxins which are taking their toll, or are we, as the proponents of the 'hygiene hypothesis' would advocate, guilty of cleaning it up so much that we reduce our exposure to pathogens and thereby affect proper development of the immune system? Much research activity is now focused on this area, but unfortunately this has not been matched by the development of new therapies.

In 1953 Sulzberger and colleagues introduced topical hydrocortisone into clinical practice thereby revolutionising treatment of atopic eczema. Topical corticosteroids have remained the mainstay of treatment for the past 50 years and their effectiveness is undoubted. Alterations to the basic molecular structure over this time have established even greater efficacy, but at the expense of an increase in adverse events. Although in many cases the risk of side-effects has been exaggerated in patients' minds, fear about them, especially in treating children, has become a deterrent to compliance with no less than 70% of patients expressing concern over their use.

Effective alternative therapy which avoids the side-effects of steroids, thereby giving a better benefit–risk ratio, is therefore badly needed. However, until recently research has been lacking. To a large extent this has been because of the absence of a clear target for therapy or indeed satisfactory models of atopic eczema, although allergic contact dermatitis is frequently used to this end. A new era in treatment is now dawning with the introduction of the topical calcineurin inhibitors. Calcineurin, an enzyme which is key in the activation of CD4 positive lymphocytes and the production of pro-inflammatory cytokines such as interleukin (IL)-2, was shown many years ago to be the main target of ciclosporin, a drug which when given systemically is highly effective in eczema but,

☞ Remember that the author of this Editorial is addressing his healthcare professional colleagues rather than the 'lay' reader. This provides a fascinating insight into many of the challenges faced by doctors in the day-to-day practice of medicine (see Reader's Guide).

because of poor absorption does not work when applied topically. Tacrolimus, which has a very different molecular structure, works in an almost identical way to ciclosporin but because of its smaller molecular weight is absorbed through the skin and is effective when used as an ointment. Pimecrolimus is a semisynthetic derivative of ascomycin, a natural fermentation product of *Streptomyces hygroscopicus* with a structure very similar to tacrolimus. Ascomycin was discovered in 1962 but not investigated further until the immunomodulatory properties of tacrolimus were discovered.

What of the future? There has been an upsurge in the introduction of new agents targeting specific cytokines in the treatment of another common skin disease, psoriasis, but with little evidence to date that they are also effective in eczema. However, further targeting the IL-2 receptor with drugs such as basiliximab might offer the possibility of potentiating the effects of calcineurin inhibitors. Although immunoglobulin E (IgE) levels are high in eczema, often higher than in asthma, there is little evidence that inhibitors of IgE activity such as omalizumab improve eczema even though they are of benefit in asthma.

Prevention is better than cure and further developments in the management of eczema are likely to develop from a better understanding of the class switch reaction. Why, for example, does a young atopic infant when presented with a common antigen switch from innate IgM to inappropriate IgE instead of the normal IgG? If we can answer this question we shall have solved the enigma of atopy.

1. Disease overview – Atopic eczema

Dr Eleanor Bull and Dr Scott Chambers
CSF Medical Communications Ltd

Summary

Atopic eczema is a chronic skin condition that presents predominantly in childhood, affecting 10–20% of school children in developed countries. The majority of cases are associated with atopy which is associated with an elevation of serum immunoglobulin E (IgE) concentrations as a result of the abnormal production of IgE antibodies in response to common environmental allergens. Symptoms of atopic eczema consist principally of dry skin and an itchy rash, often with flexural involvement, and a characteristic distribution pattern that varies with the age of the patient. Commonly, the disease first presents during early infancy and childhood but can persist into adulthood in a small proportion of patients. Atopic eczema is strongly associated with the other atopic diseases (e.g. allergic rhinitis and asthma – the so-called atopic triad), and there is some suggestion that eczema may be a precursor to the development of these other atopic conditions in later life. The clinical emergence of atopic eczema results from a combination of genetic and environmental factors. The disease is associated with higher socioeconomic class and is encountered more frequently in urban settings. The prevalence of atopic eczema has rapidly increased in recent years, particularly in the UK, Scandinavia and Japan. The 'hygiene hypothesis' relates the increased prevalence in atopic disease to reduced exposure to microbial allergens and the widespread increase in the use of antibiotics. The condition places a substantial economic burden on healthcare resources, whilst an individual patient's quality of life is severely compromised by the condition.

Introduction

Eczema denotes an inflammation of the skin, or dermatitis. It can derive from multiple causes, and its main types are atopic and contact (subdivided into allergic and irritant forms). The most common form of the condition is atopic eczema.

The term atopic describes the abnormal production of IgE antibodies in response to common environmental allergens including house-dust mites, grass, pollen, animal allergens and certain foodstuffs. Atopic eczema is a chronic inflammatory skin condition, the occurrence of which is strongly associated with other atopic diseases such as asthma and allergic rhinitis. Substantial evidence suggests that eczema may be associated with the development of these other conditions in later life. Indeed, up to 80% of children with atopic eczema will develop allergic rhinitis or asthma later in childhood.[1] There are two recognised types of atopic eczema, extrinsic, which involves IgE antibody-mediated sensitisation and affects 70–80% of the patient population, and intrinsic, which is non-IgE-mediated, affecting 20–30% of patients.[2] A highly heritable disease, atopic eczema commonly presents during early infancy and childhood, and represents the most common disease in individuals within this age group, but it may also persist into adulthood, albeit only in a proportion of patients.

Symptoms

Atopic eczema is characterised by patches of red, dry, itchy skin, often starting on the face and spreading to the outside of the limbs and body, usually in the bends of the elbows or behind the knees.

The clinical features of atopic eczema are highly variable, occurring with different skin rash morphology, in different places and over a variable time period. However, in general terms, atopic eczema is characterised by patches of red, dry, itchy skin, often starting on the face and spreading to the outside of the limbs and body, usually in the bends of the elbows or behind the knees (antecubital and popliteal fossae). Scaling and crusting on the scalp, cheeks and skin folds of the neck may also occur. Lichenification, or thickening of the skin, is normally observed in children after the ages of 3–4 years, primarily as a result of excessive and repeated scratching. In adults, exacerbations of atopic eczema are more often located on the hands. The itching, or pruritus, may worsen at night, leading to sleep deprivation, which can impact profoundly on patients' quality of life.

Atopic eczema may be complicated by recurrent viral skin infections including warts and eczema molluscatum.[3] Proliferation of *Staphylococcus aureus* may also occur on the eczematous skin of 90% of patients, a feature which may exacerbate or maintain skin inflammation and further predisposes the patient to skin infection.[4] Frequently, it leads to impetigo – lesions that develop suddenly and grow with brown crusts.[5] Occasionally, *Streptococcus pyogenes* can exacerbate eczema. Oozing from an eczematous site is an indication of infection.

Aside from the clearly visible clinical symptoms of atopic eczema, there are a number of significant psychological issues associated with the condition. As the visible manifestations of the condition commonly occur at a critical stage in the social development of a child, they may give rise to teasing and heightened self-consciousness, which may ultimately result in educational problems due to school absence and sleep deprivation.

Pathophysiology

The characteristic appearance of atopic eczema, on a microscopic level, is of excess fluid between the cells in the epidermis (spongiosis). As the build-up of fluid ensues, adjacent cells can become disrupted, leading to the formation of vesicles. Blood stem cells carrying the abnormal genetic expression of atopy, infiltrate and remain in the mucosal surfaces and the skin, leading to chronic sensitisation.[6] During the chronic phase, pruritus and associated scratching cause thickening of the epidermis (acanthosis), increased risk of infection and irritation.

Factors that contribute to atopic eczema include:
- a family history of atopy, allergic rhinitis or asthma
- IgE antibody imbalance
- microbial colonisation
- lipid and barrier impairment
- aeroallergens
- food allergy or hypersensitivity
- psychosomatic factors.[7]

There is strong evidence to show that susceptibility to atopic eczema exists in families.[8] This inheritance pattern causes cytokine gene activation and amongst the 20 or so genes implicated in atopic eczema, the locus 5q31–33, which contains the cytokine genes for interleukin (IL)-3, -4, -5, -13 and granulocyte-macrophage colony-stimulating factor (GM-CSF), appears to be particularly influential.[9] Thus, a genetic predisposition to a variety of allergenic triggers may exist in those with atopic eczema.

Immunological investigations have found that a large percentage (80–85%) of patients have an elevated serum level of IgE.[7] Heightened levels of IgE indicate an imbalance in T-cell immunity, namely, a predominance of Th2 in acute lesions. This also affects Th1 secretions of IL-2, tumour necrosis factor (TNF)-β and interferon (IFN)-γ in the chronic phase of an inflammatory response with an increased activation of macrophages, T-cell growth and monocytes. Th2 cells secrete IL-4, which stimulates IgE synthesis further. The predominance of IgE, affecting cell defences during both acute and chronic phases of disease, can lead to a higher risk of relapse from secondary fungal or viral infection.[10]

Immune stimulation resulting in skin reaction can also be caused by certain microbial organisms, for example, *S. aureus*.[11] This organism appears to be a persistent irritant with inflammatory potency on atopic skin. Studies suggest the release of superantigens, caused by the production of enterotoxins from *S. aureus*, induce marked immune stimulation.[11]

The dry, scaling skin indicative of atopic eczema suggests an impaired skin barrier function. Enhanced transepidermal water loss and reduced skin surface water content has been reported which directly reflects this theory.[12] The lipid composition within the stratum corneum, which maintains the barrier function, appears different in eczematous skin compared with normal skin.[12] This may be due, at least in part, to a metabolic abnormality. A deficiency in δ-6-desaturase, an enzyme involved in fatty acid metabolism, has been detected in atopic aczema patients.[13]

The role of food allergies in the aggravation of atopic eczema is variable in adults. Specific IgE antibodies to food, microbes and various allergens have been found (Figure 1).[14,15] Instigating dietary changes in children and infants, for instance eliminating cow's milk, seems to relieve symptoms in some cases.[7] Serum IgE levels in infants and children with atopic eczema are higher in response to food substances such as milk, nuts and wheat, compared with healthy participants.[7]

Some aeroallergens may induce eczematous skin lesions, as identified with atopy patch testing (APT). These allergens include the house-dust mite and pollen or animal dander.[16,17] Further exacerbation of symptoms in sufferers can occur from stressful emotional events. Similarly, the effects of coping with chronic disease also need to be considered.

Diagnosis

Owing to the broad and variable spectrum of its symptoms, there is no unique diagnostic test that is specific for all patients with atopic eczema. Therefore, diagnosis is largely made by the subjective assessment of the principal presenting clinical symptoms. The skin condition itself will generally exhibit exacerbations and remissions. Pruritus is the predominant feature of the condition, and, as such, a non-itching rash

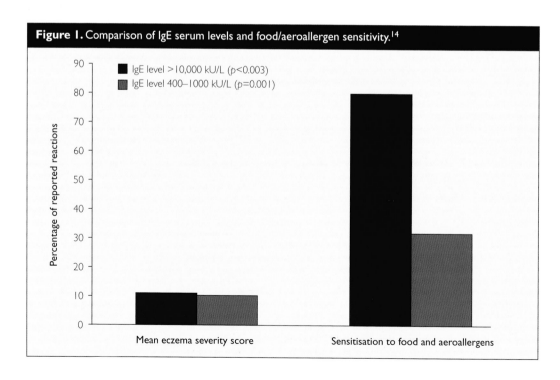

Figure 1. Comparison of IgE serum levels and food/aeroallergen sensitivity.[14]

- IgE level >10,000 kU/L (p<0.003)
- IgE level 400–1000 kU/L (p=0.001)

generally excludes a diagnosis of atopic eczema. In addition, the patient will characteristically have a family history of atopic disease.

A UK-specific revision of the Hanifin and Rajka diagnostic criteria for atopic eczema specifies a check-list of clinical symptoms.[18,19] Thus, patients with atopic eczema will have experienced an itchy skin condition in the previous 12 months, plus have evidence of three or more of the following criteria:

- onset below the age of 2 years
- past involvement of the skin creases, such as the bends of the elbows or behind the knees
- a history of generally dry skin
- personal or family history of other atopic disease
- visible flexural dermatitis.

Epidemiology

Atopic eczema is the most common disease of childhood, occurring most frequently in the first 5 years of life and affecting 10–20% of schoolchildren in Western Europe and the USA.[20,21] The prevalence in adults is much reduced, with only about 1–3% of the general population affected.[21] However, the disease tends to be more persistent and severe amongst the adult population.

The prevalence of atopic eczema has dramatically increased over the past 30 years and currently verges on epidemic proportions, for reasons that are largely unexplained.[22] In industrialised countries, in particular the UK, Scandinavia and Japan, the incidence of atopic disease has increased by two-to-three-fold over the last three decades, but it remains less common in agricultural regions including China, Eastern Europe and rural Africa.[4,23] The worldwide prevalence of atopic eczema symptoms, as determined by the International Study of Asthma and Allergies in Childhood (ISAAC) survey, is illustrated in Figure 2.[24]

> Atopic eczema is the most common disease of childhood, occurring most frequently in the first 5 years of life and affecting 10–20% of schoolchildren in Western Europe and the USA.

Aetiology

In common with the other atopic diseases, the clinical expression of atopic eczema in the individual is thought to arise from a combination of genetic and environmental factors. Whilst an individual may be genetically predisposed to atopy, it is the interaction of these factors with widespread environmental elements that may lead to the development and clinical manifestation of the disease.

Genetic components

Atopic eczema has a strong familial basis, such that the perinatal risk of developing the disease is almost double for those children with a parental history of eczema compared with those without such history.[25] Studies conducted in twins have shown that monozygotic twins have an 86% risk of having atopic eczema if the twin partner has the disease, whereas the 21% disease risk in dizygotic twins does not differ from the frequency seen in ordinary siblings.[26] As a consequence of our growing

Figure 2. Annual global prevalence of atopic eczema symptoms.[24]

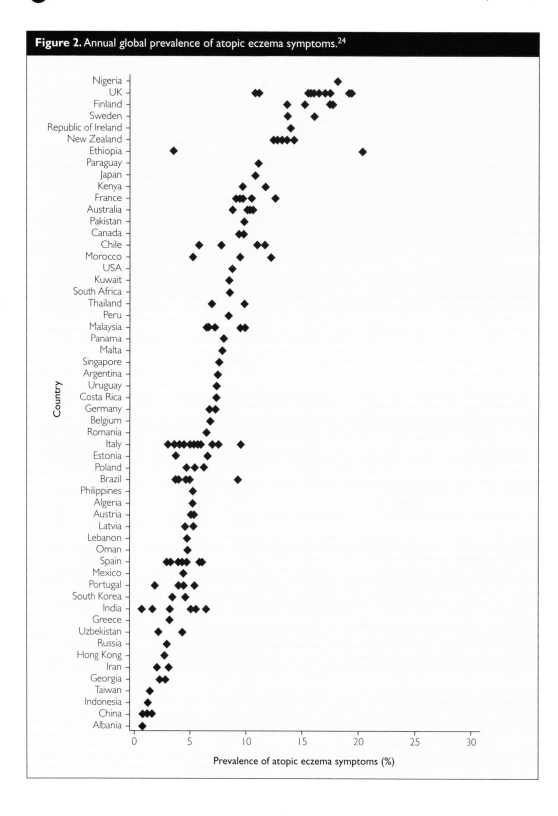

understanding of the genetic basis for the condition, the identification of specific genes underlying atopic eczema is likely within the next few years.

A US epidemiological study has reported that black or Asian race/ethnicity and male gender increase the risk of atopic eczema in the first 6 months of life.[26]

Environmental components

A number of environmental factors have also been implicated in the onset and/or exacerbation of atopic eczema. Table 1 lists some of the environmental elements which are known to contribute to disease activity. Limited evidence suggests that factors such as lower maternal age and exclusive breast-feeding during the first 3 months of life may be associated with a lower incidence of atopic eczema in children with a family history of atopy.[28]

In line with the increased incidence of atopic eczema observed in developed countries, it is thought likely that environmental factors associated with family lifestyle such as socioeconomic status, allergen exposure, family size, early childhood infections and dietary habits, may prove to be of greatest relevance. Indeed, atopic eczema is more common in wealthier families, a finding that has been linked to aspects of the home environment, including double glazing, fitted carpets, pets, increased exposure to soaps and decreased air circulation as a result of good insulation.[29] Migrant populations, moving from rural, undeveloped environments to towns and cities, exhibit increased rates of

Table 1. Factors known to contribute to disease activity in patients with atopic eczema.[5]

Physical factors
- Warm surroundings
- Physical irritation of the skin
- Climate

Psychological factors
- Stress (e.g. work related, school examinations)

Foods
- Tomato and orange juice
- Handling of certain fresh vegetables
- Juice from fish and meat

Allergens
- House-dust mites
- Animal hair and fur, pollen, plants

Other
- *Staphylococcus aureus*

atopic disease as a result of changes in allergen exposure. Overcrowding, exposure to industrial pollution, automobile exhausts, housing and bedding, central heating and eradication of parasites, may all contribute to the observed differences in disease frequency between industrialised and developing nations.[30]

The 'hygiene hypothesis' has been proposed in an attempt to rationalise the increase in the prevalence of atopic disease observed in recent years, which was not thought to be solely attributable to increases in mite and other allergen exposures.[31,32] It is based on the premise that in developed countries, an infant's immune system fails to develop appropriately as a result of reduced microbial exposure early in life in conjunction with an overuse of antibiotics, thereby increasing susceptibility to atopic disease development. The inverse association between atopic eczema and family size adds weight to this principle, by suggesting a protective effect conferred by increased cross-infection from siblings.[32]

> The 'hygiene hypothesis' has been proposed in an attempt to rationalise the increase in the prevalence of atopic disease observed in recent years.

Socioeconomic impact

Owing to its high prevalence, the management of atopic eczema exerts considerable pressure on limited public healthcare resources. Eczema-associated expenses incurred by hospitals, health authorities and individual families can be expected to increase as the frequency of the disease and cost of medication continues to rise. On the basis of prevalence estimates within the UK population, the annual personal cost (based on 1995 prices) to patients with atopic eczema has been estimated at £297 million. This is accompanied by costs to the health service of approximately £125 million, and an annual cost to society, in terms of lost schooling. The cost of lost working days has been estimated at £43 million annually.[33]

In the USA, the annual cost of treating a single patient with atopic eczema has been estimated at US$219, with costs escalating significantly with disease severity.[34] An Australian survey estimated the annual cost of treating a child with mild disease severity at Aus$1142, increasing up to Aus$6099 in those children with severe exacerbations.[34] For the parent, in addition to the personal financial cost of treatment, which exceeds that of asthma, the management of atopic eczema in a child can also result in sleep deprivation, loss of employment and emotional burden.[35,36]

Key points

- Atopic eczema is a chronic skin condition generally associated with an abnormal production of IgE antibodies in response to common environmental allergens. Most common in children, it may persist into adulthood.

- The disease is characterised by patches of red, dry itchy skin, commonly localised to the head and limbs. Lichenification of the skin and skin infections may develop as a result of the excessive scratching of affected areas.

- Major pathophysiological features include elevated serum levels of IgE and abnormal lipid composition in the skin, leading to impaired barrier function.

- Although there is usually a strong familial history of atopic disease, environmental factors, including socioeconomic status, family size, exposure to allergens and early childhood infection contribute heavily to disease manifestation.

- The increasing worldwide incidence of atopic eczema, particularly in developed countries, exerts significant pressure on healthcare resources.

References

A list of the published evidence which has been reviewed in compiling the preceding section of *BESTMEDICINE*.

1 Eichenfield L, Hanifin J, Beck L *et al.* Atopic dermatitis and asthma: parallels in the evolution of treatment. *Pediatrics* 2003; **111**: 608–16.

2 Johansson S, Hourihane J, Bousquet J *et al.* A revised nomenclature for allergy. An EAACI position statement from the EAACI nomenclature task force. *Allergy* 2001; **56**: 813–24.

3 Wollenberg A, Wetzel S, Burgdorf W, Haas J. Viral infections in atopic dermatitis: pathogenic aspects and clinical management. *J Allergy Clin Immunol* 2003; **112**: 667–74.

4 Leung D, Bieber T. Atopic dermatitis. *Lancet* 2003; **361**: 151–60.

5 Thestrup-Pedersen K. Clinical aspects of atopic dermatitis. *Clin Exp Dermatol* 2000; **25**: 535–43.

6 Hoare C, Li Wan Po A, Williams H. Systematic review of treatments for atopic eczema. *Health Technology Assessment* 2000; **4**: 13–15.

7 World Allergy Organization. Allergic Diseases Resource Center. *www.worldallergy.org*

8 Forrest S, Dunn K, Elliott K *et al.* Identifying genes predisposing to atopic eczema. *J Allergy Clin Immunol* 1999; **104**: 1066–70.

9 Schultz-Larsen F. Atopic dermatitis: a genetic-epidemiologic study in a population-based twin sample. *J Am Acad Dermatol* 1993; **28**: 719–23.

10 Hanifin J, Chan S. Biochemical and immunologic mechanisms in atopic dermatitis: new targets for emerging therapies. *J Am Acad Dermatol* 1999; **41**: 72–7.

11 Monti G, Tonetto P, Mostert M *et al.* Staphylococcus aureus skin colonization in infants with atopic dermatitis. *Dermatology* 1996; **193**: 83–7.

12 Tupker RA, Pinnagoda J, Coenraads PJ *et al.* Susceptibility to irritants: role of barrier function, skin dryness and history of atopic dermatitis. *Br J Dermatol* 1990; **123**: 199–205.

13 Horrobin DF. Fatty acid metabolism in health and disease: the role of delta-6-desaturase. *Am J Clin Nutr* 1993; **57(Suppl 5)**: 732S–36S.

14 Laske N, Bunikowski R, Niggemann B. Extraordinarily high serum IgE levels and consequences for atopic phenotypes. *Ann Allergy Asthma Immunol* 2003; **91**: 202–4.

15 Hoffman DR. Specific IgE antibodies in atopic eczema. *J Allergy Clin Immunol* 1975; **55**: 256–67.

16 Ring J, Darsow U, Gfesser M *et al.* The 'atopy patch test' in evaluating the role of aeroallergens in atopic eczema. *Int Arch Allergy Immunol* 1997; **113**: 379–83.

17 Loffler H, Steffes A, Happle R, Effendy I. Allergy and irritation: an adverse association in patients with atopic eczema. *Int Arch Allergy Immunol* 2003; **83**: 328–31.

18 Hanifin J, Rajka G. Diagnostic features of atopic dermatitis. *Acta Derm Venereol Suppl (Stockh)* 1980; **92**: 44–7.

19 Williams H. Epidemiology of atopic dermatitis. *Clin Exp Dermatol* 2000; **25**: 522–9.

20 Schultz-Larsen F, Diepgen T, Svensson A. The occurrence of atopic dermatitis in north Europe: an international questionnaire study. *J Am Acad Dermatol* 1996; **34**: 760–4.

21 Schultz-Larsen F, Hanifin J. Epidemiology of atopic dermatitis. *Immunol Allergy Clin North Am* 2002; **22**: 1–24.

22 Williams H. Is the prevalence of atopic dermatitis increasing? *Clin Exp Dermatol* 1992; **17**: 385–91.

23 Williams H, Robertson C, Stewart A *et al.* Worldwide variations in the prevalence of symptoms of atopic eczema in the International Study of Asthma and Allergies in Childhood. *J Allergy Clin Immunol* 1999; **103**: 125–38.

24 The International Study of Asthma and Allergies in Childhood. The ISAAC Steering Committee. Worldwide variation in prevalence of symptoms of asthma, allergic rhinoconjunctivitis, and atopic eczema. *Lancet* 1998; **351**: 1225–32.

25 Fergusson D, Horwood L, Shannon F. Risk factors in childhood eczema. *J Epidemiol Community Health* 1982; **36**: 118–22.

26 Larsen F, Holm N, Henningsen K. Atopic dermatitis. A genetic-epidemiologic study in a population-based twin sample. *J Am Acad Dermatol* 1986; **15**: 487–94.

27 Moore MM, Rifas-Shiman SL, Rich-Edwards JW *et al.* Perinatal predictors of atopic dermatitis occurring in the first six months of life. *Pediatrics* 2004; **113**: 468–74.

28 Gdalevich M, Mimouni D, David M, Mimouni M. Breast-feeding and the onset of atopic dermatitis in childhood: a systematic review and meta-analysis of prospective studies. *J Am Acad Dermatol* 2001; **45**: 520–7.

29 Williams H, Strachan D, Hay R. Childhood eczema: disease of the advantaged? *BMJ* 1994; **308**: 1132–5.

30 McNally N, Phillips D, Williams H. The problem of atopic eczema: aetiological clues from the environment and lifestyles. *Soc Sci Med* 1998; **46**: 729–41.

31 Strachan D. Family size, infection and atopy: the first decade of the "hygiene hypothesis". *Thorax* 2000; **55**: S2–10.

32 Strachan D. Hay fever, hygiene, and household size. *BMJ* 1989; **299**: 1259–60.

33 Herd R, Tidman M, Prescott R, Hunter J. The cost of atopic eczema. *Br J Dermatol* 1996; **135**: 20–3.

34 Weinmann S, Kamtsiuris P, Henke K, Wickman M, Jenner A, Wahn U. The costs of atopy and asthma in children: assessment of direct costs and their determinants in a birth cohort. *Pediatr Allergy Immunol* 2003; **14**: 18–26.

35 Kemp A. Atopic eczema: its social and financial costs. *J Paediatr Child Health* 1999; **35**: 229–31.

36 Su J, Kemp A, Varigos G, Nolan T. Atopic eczema: its impact on the family and financial cost. *Arch Dis Child* 1997; **76**: 159–62.

Acknowledgements

Figure 2 is adapted from ISAAC, 1998.[24]

2. Management options – Atopic eczema

Dr Rebecca Fox-Spencer
CSF Medical Communications Ltd

Summary

The management of atopic eczema focuses on minimising the impact
that persistent symptoms and exacerbations of the disease can have
on a patient's quality of life. The recently licensed topical
immunosuppressant drugs – the main focus of this edition of
BESTMEDICINE – have complemented the wide array of treatment
options currently available for atopic eczema. Topical corticosteroids
are used to treat exacerbations of atopic eczema, whereas
emollients provide a prophylactic skin care option. Together, these
two treatments are considered to be the first-line management
strategy for the condition, though there is very little clinical data
available to support the use of emollients. Depending on the
presentation of the condition, these conventional options may be
supplemented with additional treatments such as antibiotics and
antipruritic agents. Dietary supplementation is a strategy adopted by
some patients, and a number of lifestyle modifications are also
recommended. Although some of these changes are supported by
clinical evidence, some may require considerable and perhaps
unreasonable commitment and effort on the part of the patient or, in
the case of a child, their parents. Finally, complementary and
alternative medicine options, including homeopathy and massage, are
used by many patients, though there is very little definitive evidence
to show that these strategies are effective. Chinese traditional
medicine is another relatively popular choice, but safety concerns
persist about the nature of this approach.

Therapeutic objectives

Given that there is no current cure for atopic eczema, the management
of the disease is focused on keeping it under control and minimising its
impact on patients' quality of life. The objectives of treatment are to:

- reduce signs and symptoms
- prevent or reduce disease recurrence
- provide long-term management by preventing exacerbation
- modify the course of the disease.[1]

Effective management of atopic eczema incorporates both treatment options and lifestyle modification. A summary of the guidelines for the management of atopic eczema issued by the Primary Care Dermatology Society and the British Association of Dermatologists is shown in Box 1.[2] Treatment options range from targeted pharmacological therapies, for which efficacy has been demonstrated in robust clinical trials, through general skin care strategies, to complementary medicines, for which there is very little supporting scientific evidence. The selection of management options depends very much on the individual patient and the features of their disease.

Topical corticosteroids

Topical corticosteroids (steroids) have long represented the first-line pharmacological treatment option for flare-ups (exacerbations) of atopic eczema, due to their suppressive effects on inflammation and pruritus.[3] Indeed, this drug class has been used for treatment of eczema for the last 40 years. During this time, the range of topical corticosteroids available for use in atopic eczema has expanded to include drugs with a wide range of potencies (Table 1). This enables the choice of corticosteroid to be tailored to the severity of the disease, the age of the patient and the area of the body to be treated (many corticosteroids are not indicated for use in more sensitive areas such as the face and flexures). This approach would be expected to aid patient compliance, given the (often exaggerated) fears associated with higher potency steroid treatment. Children are particularly susceptible to the side-effects of corticosteroids, thus the use of these drugs should be restricted to mild formulations as long as this enables adequate control of the condition.[4] Moderately potent or potent corticosteroids may be used to treat severe atopic eczema on the limbs of children, but only for 1–2 weeks.

The range of drugs is sufficiently diverse to have prompted the comment that the market is currently 'saturated' with many different strengths and formulations of topical corticosteroids.[5] As indicated in Table 1, most of these drugs are also available in more than one formulation, enabling the choice of treatment to be further tailored to the skin condition of the individual patient. Whereas creams are more suitable for lesions which are moist or weeping, ointments are more useful for lesions which are dry or scaly, as they have a more occlusive effect. In contrast, lotions are best suited to larger or hairy regions, or for the treatment of weeping lesions. Administration of topical corticosteroids under occlusion improves their absorption into the skin. Various methods are available for occlusive drug administration, but these should be reserved for short treatment durations on regions of

> Effective management of atopic eczema incorporates both treatment options and lifestyle modification.

> The range of topical corticosteroids available for use in atopic eczema has expanded to include drugs with a wide range of potencies.

Box 1. Summary of guidelines for the management of atopic eczema, issued by the Primary Care Dermatology Society and the British Association of Dermatologists.[2]

General principles of primary care management:
- Keep the patient/parent informed and educated.
- Whilst appreciating the practical limitations, advise the patient to avoid exacerbating factors.
- Advise the patient on how to keep skin hydrated.
- Treat secondary infection early.
- Treat exacerbations with acute topical steroids.

Use of emollients:
- Most patients require general use of emollients.
- Should be applied as liberally and frequently as possible, particularly when skin is moist.
- Should exceed corticosteroid use by approximately 10:1.
- Complete emollient therapy (cream, ointment, bath oil and soap substitute) will aid maximum effect.
- If applied after a topical corticosteroid, ideally delay for at least 30 minutes.
- Emollients may be supplemented with antipruritic or antiseptic agents.

Use of topical corticosteroids:
- Topical steroids are safe in the short term, the weakest drug which effectively controls symptoms should be used.
- Limit treatment to a few days a week for acute eczema, up to 4–6 weeks for initial remission in chronic eczema.
- Review potency and quantity of steroid used on a regular basis.
- Patients using moderate or potent steroids must be monitored closely for local and systemic side-effects. Very potent steroids, particularly in children, should generally only be used on the advice of a specialist.

Use of topical immunomodulatory agents:
- New alternative to topical corticosteroids, though generally more expensive and no more effective.
- Only to be considered for patients intolerant to, or not responsive to, topical corticosteroids.
- Should be initiated by a specialist, with advice offered on photoprotection.

Management of bacterial infection:
- Oral antibiotics often necessary in moderate-to-severe infection.
- Corticosteroid-antibiotic combinations available.
- Swabs for bacteriology useful if patients do not respond to treatment.
- Advise patient on general measures to avoid infection.

Alternative treatments:
- Antihistamines.
- Phototherapy.
- Various immunosuppressive agents.

Table 1. Topical corticosteroids licensed for the treatment of atopic eczema in the UK. For simplicity, preparations including active ingredients other than corticosteroids are excluded from this table (see footnotes).[4]

Agent	Trade name	Formulation	Concentration (%)
Mild potency			
Hydrocortisone (all forms except for hydrocortisone butyrate)[a]	Non-proprietary formulations; Dermacort®; Zenoxone®; Dioderm®; Efcortelan®; Mildison®; Hc45®; Lanacort®;	Cream and ointment	0.1, 0.25, 0.5, 1
Fluocinolone acetonide	Synalar 1 in 10 dilution®	Cream	0.0025
Moderate potency			
Alclometasone dipropionate	Modrasone®	Cream and ointment	0.05
Betamethasone esters	Betnovate-RD®	Cream and ointment	0.025
Clobetasone butyrate[b]	Eumovate®	Cream and ointment	0.05
Fludroxycortide	Haelan®	Cream, ointment and tape	0.0125
Fluocinolone acetonide	Synalar® (1 in 4 dilution)	Cream and ointment	0.00625
Fluocortolone	Ultralanum plain®	Cream and ointment	0.25
Potent			
Hydrocortisone butyrate[b]	Locoid®, Locoid Crelo®, Locoid C®	Cream, ointment and lotion	0.1
Beclometasone dipropionate	Propaderm®	Cream and ointment	0.025
Betamethasone esters[c]	Non-proprietary; Betacap®; Betnovate®; Bettamousse®; Diprosone®	Cream, ointment, foam, lotion, scalp application	0.05, 0.1
Diflucortolone valerate	Nerisone®	Cream and ointment	0.1
Fluocinolone acetonide[e]	Synalar®	Cream, ointment and gel	0.025
Fluocinolide	Metosyn®	Cream and ointment	0.05
Fluticasone propionate	Cutivate®	Cream and ointment	0.005, 0.05
Mometasone furoate	Elocon®	Cream, ointment and lotion	0.1
Very potent			
Clobetasol propionate[b]	Dermovate®	Cream, ointment and scalp application	0.05
Diflucortolone valerate	Nerisone Forte®	Cream and ointment	0.3
Halcinonide	Halciderm Topical®	Cream	0.1

[a]available in compound preparations with coal tar, antimicrobials or crotamiton; [b]available in compound preparations with antimicrobials; [c]available in compound preparations with salicylic acid or with antimicrobials; [d]available as a lotion compound preparation with salicylic acid; [e]available in compound preparations with antibacterials.
N.B. triamcinolone acetonide is only available with antimicrobials.

thick skin, due to the associated risk of adverse events.[4] Occlusive techniques, such as wet wrap therapy, described later in this review, are generally prescribed only by specialists.

Mechanism of action

Topical corticosteroids act by modulating gene expression within epidermal and dermal cells, as well as leukocytes that participate in cutaneous inflammatory reactions. Corticosteroids bind to specific receptors within these cells, and then the steroid–receptor complexes translocate to the cell nuclei, where they bind to 'glucocorticoid response elements' within the DNA (Figure 1). This binding alters the level of transcription of messenger RNA (mRNA), in turn modulating the synthesis of proteins involved in the inflammatory process.[6,7]

Clinical evidence

Given that the use of topical corticosteroids for the treatment of atopic eczema is so well established in clinical practice, there is a surprising paucity of good quality clinical trial data demonstrating the efficacy of these drugs in this setting.

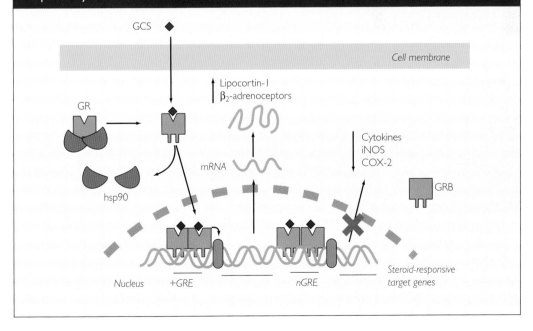

Figure 1. Mechanism of action of corticosteroids.[7] The steroid molecule (GCS) enters the cell and binds to a cytoplasmic glucocorticoid receptor (GR) that is complexed with two molecules of a heat shock protein (hsp90). The steroid–GR complex translocates to the nucleus, where it binds to the glucocorticoid response element (GRE) located on glucocorticoid-responsive genes. GREs may increase transcription and negative (n)GREs may decrease transcription, resulting in increased or decreased mRNA and protein synthesis.

A large systematic review of treatments for atopic eczema initially identified a total of 83 randomised controlled trials which gave a sufficiently clear description of the patient population and presented results from patients with atopic eczema separately from those with other inflammatory dermatoses.[5] However, of these trials, only 13 compared topical corticosteroids with placebo, and none included betamethasone valerate, despite its use as a standard comparator for most newly developed corticosteroids. In addition, the quality of many of these studies was considered poor, of only short duration and with a strong emphasis placed on subjective patient-rated outcomes. Despite these limitations, these trials did report a large effect of corticosteroid treatment. Studies reporting comparisons within the drug class were more common (n=40) but again were often of poor quality.

As indicated in Table 1, a number of the topical corticosteroids available in the UK are available as compound preparations combined with crotamiton, coal tar, salicylic acid or antimicrobials. Crotamiton is an antipruritic agent, whilst coal tar is reported to exhibit both anti-inflammatory and antiscaling properties.[4] The inclusion of salicylic acid increases the penetration of the drug, as well as offering weak antimicrobial properties.[4] Topical triamcinolone acetonide is only available as a compound treatment with antimicrobials. Secondary skin infections, particularly by *Staphylococcus aureus*, are common in patients with atopic eczema. *S. aureus* can be isolated from skin lesions of most patients with atopic eczema. By contrast, these bacteria colonise the skin of less than 5% of non-eczematous individuals.[8] The association between eczema and infection is thought to arise partly because of the enhanced avidity of inflamed atopic skin for *S. aureus*, as well as a reduced expression of antimicrobial peptides in these individuals. Infection can further promote inflammation and alter the sensitivity to therapy. The use of corticosteroid–antimicrobial compound therapies would therefore appear to be a sensible treatment strategy in patients with secondary infection. These combination drugs are widely used, though there is no data from clinical trials to suggest that treatment of the infection in this way confers any additional improvement to patients' eczema.[5] Three randomised controlled trials have compared corticosteroid–antimicrobial compound treatments with corticosteroid treatment alone, and have demonstrated no significant additional benefit in terms of the severity of eczema.[9–11]

Useful data have been obtained from a retrospective analysis of clinical data from 1271 patients with atopic eczema in Japan.[12] Although this was not a controlled analysis and patients had a variety of treatment histories, the data clearly demonstrated that a substantial proportion of patients were not satisfactorily treated with topical corticosteroids. In 7% of infantile cases, 10% of childhood cases and 19% of adolescent and adult cases, patients remained in a 'severe' or 'very severe' state or experienced further exacerbations following 6 months of treatment with corticosteroids. There was a trend for patients whose condition was considered 'uncontrolled' to be using milder corticosteroids, whilst patients whose symptoms were considered well controlled were receiving more potent drugs. Adjustments of dose

> Three randomised controlled trials have compared corticosteroid–antimicrobial compound treatments with corticosteroid treatment alone, and have demonstrated no significant additional benefit in terms of the severity of eczema.

and potency of topical steroids are therefore important in the management of atopic eczema. Reluctance on the part of patients or physicians to make these adjustments is a significant limitation to the effectiveness of corticosteroids in clinical practice.

Safety and tolerability

Compliance to treatment is further complicated by the chronic nature of the condition, which demands long-term treatment. There are a number of concerns regarding the long-term use of topical steroids in managing atopic eczema. Guidelines recommend that corticosteroid use should be limited to only a few days a week for acute eczema, and up to 4–6 weeks to gain initial remission from chronic eczema.[2] Care should be taken in selecting the appropriate drug potency for each individual patient.

The most common local side-effect associated with the topical corticosteroids is skin atrophy, which results from their suppressive effects on connective tissue. The risk of atrophy is particularly high in regions such as the face and flexures, where the skin is already thin.[13] For this reason, repeated application of topical steroids is not recommended in these regions, whilst the use of more potent drugs should generally be avoided.[2,13] The risk of steroid-induced skin atrophy is also increased if the drug is applied under occlusion. Although most cases of skin atrophy are mild and reversible, profound cases may induce striae atrophica (stretch marks), which is a more serious and irreversible side-effect.[12] Additional steroid-related side-effects include contact dermatitis, telangiectasia, acne, mild depigmentation and spread or worsening of untreated infection.[4] There is also a further risk associated with the use of these drugs on the eyelids, as contamination of the conjunctiva can lead to glaucoma simplex or subcapsular cataract.

Much of the concern over the safety profile of corticosteroids is related to the systemic effects of these drugs, which include suppression of the hypothalamic–pituitary–adrenal (HPA) axis, leading to growth retardation and/or Cushing's syndrome. The risk of these effects depends upon the potency of the corticosteroid used, the extent of drug exposure (based on the size of the body area affected and the duration of application) and the age of the patient. Children and infants are most susceptible to the systemic effects of corticosteroids due to their relatively large surface area-to-body weight ratio. It is, therefore, strongly recommended that the use of moderately potent topical corticosteroids by these patients is monitored carefully by a specialist. In adults, the risks of systemic adverse events can be minimised by adhering to recommended dose limits, according to the potency of the drug and the intended duration of its use (Table 2).[14]

In summary, the safety concerns associated with topical steroids can be minimised by limiting the potency of the drug selected and by restricting treatment periods to short bursts, in response to flare-ups and not as a prophylactic therapy. Although these drugs are generally recommended for application 1–2-times daily,[4] several studies have suggested that increasing the frequency of application to more than once daily does not enhance efficacy.[15]

> The most common local side-effect of treatment with topical corticosteroids is skin atrophy, which results from their suppressive effects on connective tissue.

> The safety issues associated with topical steroids can be minimised by limiting the potency of the drug selected and by restricting treatment periods to short bursts.

Table 2. Weekly dose of corticosteroids considered unlikely to cause systemic adverse events in adults.[14]

Treatment period (months)	Mild and moderately potent	Potent	Very potent
<2 months	100 g	50 g	30 g
2–6 months	50 g	30 g	15 g
6–12 months	25 g	15 g	7.5 g

Pharmacoeconomics

There are very limited pharmacoeconomic data available regarding the use of topical corticosteroids in atopic eczema. Cost-effectiveness analyses are confounded by the variability in the quantity of drug used per application and the frequency of flare-ups necessitating treatment.[13] Clearly, once-daily application has lower direct costs than twice-daily administration. In addition, the wide array of steroids available has also driven down costs. Consequently, guidelines recommend that when more than one topical steroid is appropriate for treatment, the product with the lowest acquisition cost (bearing in mind the pack size and advised frequency of application) should be used in preference.[13]

Conclusion

In conclusion, topical corticosteroids have long been considered the first-line option for pharmacological management of flare-ups in atopic eczema, and this remains the case despite the introduction of the topical immunomodulators. However, in patients whose condition is not adequately controlled with corticosteroid therapy, or those whom adverse events cause major tolerability issues, the use of topical immunomodulatory agents may be more appropriate.[2]

Emollients

Although topical corticosteroids are recommended as the first-line treatment option for flare-ups of atopic eczema, the main prophylactic strategy lies in good skin care.[2] Atopic eczema is characterised by dry skin, which is not just a secondary phenomenon, but a critical exacerbant of the condition, and a major recognised cause of pruritus. Furthermore, skin dryness can lead to inflammation.[5] When the barrier properties of the skin are defective, susceptibility to irritants or allergens is increased, as is the potential for transepidermal water loss, which accentuates the problem (Figure 2).[16]

Atopic eczema is characterised by dry skin, which is not just a secondary phenomenon, but a critical exacerbant of the condition.

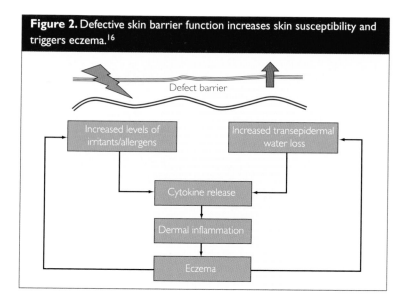

Figure 2. Defective skin barrier function increases skin susceptibility and triggers eczema.[16]

Mechanism of action

The stratum corneum (the outermost layer of the epidermis) requires a water content of at least 10% for its normal appearance and function, but in patients with atopic eczema it is less hydrated and less capable of binding water. In eczematous skin, there is an increased number of cell layers in the stratum corneum, with increased cohesion between them. Eczematous skin is also characterised by an abnormal lipid composition, including a reduction in the amount of ceramides, altered distribution of ceramide types and elevated cholesterol. These properties reduce the barrier function of the skin and make it less supple.[16]

These morphological features appear to be normalised to some extent by the regular use of emollients or moisturisers. Although these two terms are often used synonymously, an emollient is technically defined as any material which softens or smoothes the skin, whereas the term 'moisturiser' implies the specific addition of water to the skin.[16] As well as relieving visible signs of dryness, these treatments provide some restoration to the barrier function of the skin. Moisturisers increase skin hydration by physically occluding the skin surface, as well as through the action of ingredients (known as humectants), which enhance the water-binding capacity of the stratum corneum. The resulting increase in hydration improves its elasticity, as well as reducing the risk of cracking, and therefore further barrier disruption. The oils, lotions, creams and ointments prescribed by physicians for good skin care are generally described as emollients rather than moisturisers, though some contain urea as a hydrating agent (Table 3).[4] It is recommended that these agents are applied at least three-times daily, and especially after bathing or taking a shower.[14]

> An emollient is technically defined as any material which softens or smoothes the skin, whereas the term 'moisturiser' implies the specific addition of water to the skin.

Table 3. Emollients prescribed in the UK.[4]

Non-proprietary preparations	Proprietary preparations	Preparations containing urea as a hydrating agent	Preparations containing antimicrobials	Bath additives
Aqueous cream, BP	Aveeno®	Aquadrate®	Dermol®	Alpha Keri Bath®
Emulsifying ointment, BP	Cetraben® Emollient Cream	Balneum® Plus		Aveeno®
Hydrous ointment, BP	Decubal® Clinic	Calmurid®		Balneum®
Liquid and white soft paraffin ointment, NPF	Dermamist®	E45® Itch Relief Cream		Cetraben®
Paraffin, white soft, BP	Diprobase®	Eucerin®		Dermalo®
Paraffin, yellow soft, BP	Doublebase®	Nutraplus®		Dermol®a
	Drapolene®			Diprobath®
	E45®			E45®
	Epaderm®			Emollient Medicinal Bath Oil
	Gammaderm®			Emulsiderm®a
	Hewletts Cream®			Hydromol Emollient®
	Hydromol®			Imuderm®
	Kamillosan®			Oilatum®b
	Keri®			
	LactiCare®			
	Lipobase®			
	Neutrogena® Dermatological Cream			
	Oilatum®			
	Ultrabase®			
	Unguentum M®			
	Vaseline Dermacare®			
	Zerobase®			

acontains antimicrobials.
bavailable with or without antimicrobials.
BP, British Pharmacopoeia; NPF, Nurse Prescribers' Formulary.

Emollients have varying lipid contents, with the lipid-to-water ratio being lowest in lotions, intermediate in creams and highest in ointments.[14] Certain lipids are thought to penetrate into the skin and normalise the endogenous lipid composition.[16] Furthermore, a number of lipids, such as essential fatty acids (e.g. linoleic acid), are thought to exhibit anti-inflammatory properties, which may contribute to their benefits in atopic eczema.

Clinical evidence

Although widely used, and indeed the most universally recommended preventative therapy for atopic eczema in the UK, there are very few data demonstrating the efficacy of emollients in a controlled trial setting.[5] An assessment of the prophylactic value of a fatty-acid rich emollient cream has demonstrated a significantly reduced response on an 'atopy patch test' following pre-treatment of the test site with the emollient.[17] In a randomised controlled trial, the emollient Cetaphil® (not available in the UK) was applied three-times daily by patients already receiving a twice-daily topical corticosteroid, and the symptoms and signs of atopic eczema in these patients were compared with those who continued on corticosteroids alone.[18] After 3 weeks, total symptom scores were reduced by 80% in those applying the emollient, compared with 70% in those who did not ($p<0.01$).

The benefits of adding urea to emollients have been assessed in a randomised controlled trial.[19] This study demonstrated that the inclusion of urea significantly increased skin hydration compared with when the emollient was given alone, and this translated to reductions in skin redness and induration. Similarly, the inclusion of ammonium lactate has been shown to be slightly more effective than an emollient alone in terms of reducing lichenification, hyperkeratosis and dryness.[20]

> There are very few data demonstrating the efficacy of emollients in a controlled trial setting.

Safety and tolerability

Mild adverse skin reactions following application of emollients or moisturisers are not uncommon, with smarting, burning and stinging sensations the most frequently reported.[16] As is the case with other topical treatments for atopic eczema, the excipients used in emollient formulations (e.g. alcohol, fragrances, wool fat, lanolin) may prove to be sensitising agents, though in practice this appears to be rare. Many available moisturising skin products are not aimed specifically at atopic individuals, and fragrances are often included in order to improve acceptability. Arachis (peanut) oil is used as an emollient agent in a number of proprietary preparations, and may be associated with the development of peanut allergy in some patients.[4,21] Rarely, emollients may cause cosmetic acne or folliculitis due to physical obstruction of the follicular orifices. Similarly, thick formulations can block sweat gland orifices in hot weather, leading to heat rash. Systemic adverse events are extremely rare, and are thought to result from excessive application of supplementary components such as salicylic acid or propylene glycol

> Mild adverse skin reactions following application of emollients or moisturisers are not uncommon, with smarting, burning and stinging sensations the most frequently reported.

rather than the emollient itself.[16] Finally, the use of emollient bath additives carries the increased risk of accidents from slipping.[5]

Conclusion

Although the rationale for the use of emollients as a prophylactic therapy in atopic eczema is clear, the clinical evidence in support of their efficacy is extremely limited. In particular, claims that these formulations have a 'steroid-sparing effect' remain largely unsubstantiated. Given the widespread use of emollients and the costs associated with this practice, there is increasing demand for robust demonstration of their value.[5]

Topical immunomodulators

The most recent development in treatment options for atopic eczema is the introduction of topical immunomodulators (alternatively called calcineurin inhibitors). Two drugs in this class are currently available in the UK: pimecrolimus (Elidel®), for acute treatment of mild-to-moderate atopic eczema, and tacrolimus (Protopic®), for use in moderate-to-severe atopic eczema which is unresponsive to other therapy.[4] By inhibiting the phosphatase enzyme, calcineurin, these drugs act to down-regulate the immune response locally at the site of topical application.[22] They also offer a non-steroidal means by which to inhibit the inflammation associated with atopic eczema. Clinical trials have demonstrated that these drugs are effective and well tolerated in adults and children over the age of 2 years, with the principal side-effect reported to be a local irritation at the application site, commonly described as a burning sensation.[23–25]

> The most recent development in treatment options for atopic eczema is the introduction of topical immunomodulators.

As the latest addition to a wide spectrum of treatment options, these two drugs are the focus of the detailed drug reviews that are included in this edition of *BESTMEDICINE*.

Secondary treatment options

Antipruritic agents

The oral H_1-receptor antagonists (e.g. levocetirizine, fexofenadine and loratadine) block the activation of H_1-receptors located on dermal mast cells and may relieve histamine-mediated aspects of the itch response. Consequently, these compounds are of limited value if the cause of the itch is not histamine-related. Indeed, two randomised controlled trials investigating the antipruritic properties of two antihistamines – chlorpheniramine and cetirizine – reported no significant reduction in pruritus compared with placebo.[26,27] These studies were conducted in children under the age of 12 years with atopic eczema. However, the central sedative effects of certain H_1-receptor antagonists such as chloramphenamine may help to avoid the sleep deprivation associated with eczema-related itch.

> The central sedative effects of certain H_1-receptor antagonists such as chloramphenamine may help to avoid the sleep deprivation associated with eczema-related itch.

Other treatments such as ichthammol paste and coal tar may be used, particularly in medicated bandages, to relieve itch. However, the use of coal tar is no longer recommended because of its unpleasant odour, potential for staining and its irritant effects on broken skin.

Antimicrobials

Secondary bacterial infection is common in patients with atopic eczema.[8] The use of antibiotics (e.g. erythromycin, flucloxacillin, azithromycin, clarithromycin, dicloxacillin and oxacillin) is advocated in patients with poorly controlled atopic eczema or in those displaying signs of clinical infection of scratched or broken skin, often due to the bacterium *S. aureus*. Antimicrobials are also often administered in compound preparations with topical corticosteroids. A bacterial skin swab may guide the clinician as to the nature of the pathogen and any antibiotic sensitivities which may exist. Atopic patients are also more susceptible to viral infections than non-atopic individuals. The most clinically relevant of these viral infections is eczema herpeticum, a disseminated infection of atopic eczema by the herpes simplex virus.[28] Systemic antiviral chemotherapy may be used to combat this infection, which is potentially life-threatening, and particularly dangerous in children.

Probiotics

Given that epidemiological data supports an inverse relationship between infection and atopy, there may be a rationale for using probiotics in the management of the condition in young infants.[29] Specific microbial agents are understood to counter-regulate atopic immune responses. Consumption of certain microbial agents has been shown to reduce the extent, severity and symptoms of atopic eczema in young infants.[29]

Systemic immunomodulation

Ciclosporin shares a similar mechanism of action with the topical immunomodulators, tacrolimus and pimecrolimus, and inhibits the phosphatase enzyme calcineurin, thus blocking the generation of inflammatory cytokines from activated T lymphocytes. Ciclosporin is not active topically, and is therefore administered orally. It is a potent immunosuppressor, and as such is only indicated for patients over the age of 16 years with severe eczema, for short-term treatment periods (maximum of 8 weeks) only.[4] Ciclosporin has a range of side-effects, including raised serum creatinine, renal impairment, hypertension and a 'rebound effect' upon symptoms following treatment discontinuation.[30] Ciclosporin is contraindicated in patients with abnormal renal function, uncontrolled hypertension, uncontrolled infections and malignancy. It is not recommended for use in patients undergoing ultraviolet (UV)-radiation phototherapy, and patients should avoid excessive exposure to sunlight during treatment.[4]

Phototherapy

UV-radiation therapy has been used for many years to treat atopic eczema and other common skin diseases, though it is not a major treatment strategy in current clinical practice.[2] Treatment may use UV-A (closest in wavelength to visible light), UV-B (lower wavelength, more strongly associated with tanning, sunburn and skin cancer) or a combination of both.[5] The mechanisms by which UV phototherapy reduces symptoms of atopic eczema are unclear, but UV-B is known to have immunosuppressive properties, whilst UV-A promotes apoptosis of inflammatory cells by means of free radical production.[5,31] However, there is little consensus over whether UV-A, UV-B, or the combination is the most effective therapy.[5,31] An additional UV-radiation option is PUVA, a combination of UV-A and psoralen, which is a photoactive drug taken either orally or mixed in a bath, and acts to enhance the effectiveness of UV-A radiation.

Although these treatments are considered to be relatively safe, long-term multicentre surveillance studies are required in large patient populations to establish whether there is a subsequent risk of skin cancer. UV radiation is a well-known carcinogen, and therefore its long-term use is not advised in children or young adults, nor in patients who are also receiving immunosuppressive treatment, as is often the case in those with atopic eczema.[32] In terms of immediate adverse events, stinging has been reported, which may be alleviated by the use of air conditioning. However, there have also been reports of more severe burning. The oral psoralen component of PUVA has been associated with occasional gastrointestinal intolerance.[5,31]

Phototherapy with UV-free radiation may also be of potential value in the management of atopic eczema.[32] It has been shown that light in the visible range can generate free radicals in the same way as UV-A, and furthermore, can induce significant improvements in eczema severity after only four treatments. In addition, improvements at non-irradiated sites were also reported, suggesting that there may be some systemic effect associated with this technique. This treatment strategy is still in its infancy, but may supersede UV-based methods in the interests of safety.

Wet wrap therapy

This strategy is used widely by specialists in the UK, particularly for treating atopic eczema in children.[14] The technique acts not only to provide a physical barrier to scratching, but also to improve absorption of emollients or topical corticosteroids, and to cool and soothe the skin. The most common method of applying a wet wrap is to coat the skin with emollient or corticosteroid, and then to wrap it in bandages which have been soaked in warm water. They are generally only used when other treatments have failed, and for short periods, often overnight. Whilst this approach is highly effective in some patients, there is concern that its use should be more closely regulated.[33] This is consistent with use of the technique being restricted to specialist care.[14] The use of

> UV radiation is a well-known carcinogen, and therefore its long-term use is not advised in children or young adults, nor in patients who are also receiving immunosuppressive treatment.

> The use of topical corticosteroids under occlusion increases the risk of systemic absorption.

topical corticosteroids under occlusion increases the risk of systemic absorption, and hence the associated risks of growth retardation and other adverse events associated with the suppression of the HPA axis.

Complementary and alternative medicine

Traditional Chinese medicine

Traditional Chinese medicine uses a combination of acupuncture, herbs, dietary manipulation and Tai Chi exercise for the prevention and treatment of a variety of illnesses and diseases, with the focus on maintaining a balance of body, mind and environment.[34] There are indications that such approaches may have anti-inflammatory and immunosuppressive properties, as well as antibacterial, antifungal, antihistaminic and muscle-relaxant effects, and thus are of potential benefit in managing atopic eczema.[35] Indeed, it is a common choice by eczematous patients.[35]

A confounding factor in the formal clinical testing of traditional Chinese medicine is the fact that standardisation of herbal mixtures contradicts the philosophy of the technique – each mixture should be individually tailored to the patient in question. In compromise, however, a standardised mixture of herbs known as Zemaphyte has been evaluated in clinical trials. A systematic review has analysed data derived from four such trials and has reported some benefits of Zemaphyte treatment, though the findings were inconsistent between the trials.[34] The studies with positive results were subject to relatively high drop-out rates, and the data reflected only those who remained in the trials, and therefore it is likely that there was a 'withdrawal bias' towards positive results. Only a small number of adverse events were reported during treatment, though a follow-up study has revealed a worrying association with abnormal liver function. These four studies were small, and considered to be of poor quality. The findings of this systematic review are consistent with the failure of the manufacturer to obtain a license of Zemaphyte for the treatment of atopic eczema.[34]

Although these controlled trials have failed to demonstrate a robust and repeatable benefit of traditional Chinese medicine in patients with atopic eczema, the use of this technique in a more traditional setting, without standardisation of the herbal mixture, has been shown to be an efficient treatment modality.[35] However, with no regulation of the composition of these remedies, concern persists over reports of contamination with toxins such as heavy metals, and indeed drugs such as corticosteroids, diazepam, phenylbutazone, paracetamol and thiamine. As such, the benefits associated with Chinese traditional medicines may possibly be associated with their corticosteroid content. The unregulated inclusion of such drugs most likely contributes to the poor safety profile of these medicines, amid reports of hypersensitivity, hepato- and nephrotoxicity, agranulocytosis, cardiomyopathy, respiratory distress syndrome and even death.[35] Furthermore, traditional Chinese medicine is not advised in pregnancy, nor in those with pre-existing liver,

The unregulated inclusion of drugs most likely contributes to the poor safety profile of these medicines.

kidney or cardiac disease. Compliance to traditional Chinese medicine is also limited by the complicated preparation techniques and the unpleasant taste of the herbal mixtures.

Acupuncture is amongst the better regulated components of Chinese traditional medicine, and its use within the NHS is growing more quickly than any other complementary therapy.[36] There is a clear lack of controlled studies concerning the effectiveness of this strategy in the management of atopic eczema compared with placebo, though it is considered to be safe if carried out by a trained practitioner. There are various forms of acupuncture available, including non-needle versions such as transcutaneous electrical nerve stimulation.[37]

Homeopathy

The practice of homeopathy involves the administration of an agent, known to cause the relevant symptoms in a healthy individual, in a hugely diluted form, with the underlying principle that the higher the dilution, the greater the effect. Until recently, homeopathic techniques have not been subjected to robust clinical testing.[38] In the last two decades, however, homeopathists have become more willing to engage in such trials. To date, randomised, double-blind trials of homeopathy in dermatological conditions have demonstrated no positive, reproducible effects. It appears likely that changes previously identified in trials which were not placebo-controlled reflected only the natural course of the disease. Furthermore, homeopathy has been associated with indirect side-effects due to withdrawal of an effective treatment. It must be conceded that an absence of robust clinical data is a feature shared with a number of more well-established treatment options for atopic eczema (e.g. emollients). However, the benefits of homeopathic treatment would appear to rest mainly in the emotional well-being of the patient, due to the opportunity, for example, to adopt a more proactive role in the choice of how to manage their condition.[38]

> To date, randomised, double-blind trials of homeopathy in dermatological conditions have demonstrated no positive, reproducible effects.

Massage/aromatherapy

A trial investigating the use of massage in young children demonstrated benefits in terms of anxiety, tactile defensiveness and ability to cope with their disease.[39] Although unlikely to be an effect specifically beneficial to eczema symptoms, the use of massage may be advantageous from a psychological perspective. In a separate trial, the combination of massage and counselling afforded benefits in terms of daytime irritation and night-time disturbance scores, as well as general disease improvement scores, in patients aged 3–7 years.[40] There was no additional advantage, however, associated with the use of aromatherapy essential oils.

Dietary supplementation

Alterations in the metabolism of linoleic acid to linolenic acid have been demonstrated in some patients with atopic eczema. As a consequence, dietary supplementation with essential fatty acids has been used in an attempt to normalise the disrupted lipid barrier in atopic skin. Linolenic acid may be administered in the form of evening primrose oil (8–10% γ-linolenic acid, also available in topical form) or in borage oil (at least 23% γ-linolenic acid). There are no consistently reported benefits associated with the use of these supplements in a clinical trial setting, though there have been claims of moderate improvement.[5] Fish oils are also rich in fatty acids, but again there is little evidence from clinical trials to support their use as a dietary supplement in patients with atopic eczema.[5]

Other dietary supplements assessed for their value in atopic eczema include vitamin E and multivitamins, as well as zinc salts. None of these has been demonstrated to benefit patients in robust, well-designed trials. Although most likely to be a chance effect, one study reported that multivitamin supplementation in early pregnancy was associated with an increased risk of atopic eczema in the child.

> There are no consistently reported benefits associated with the use of dietary linolenic acid supplements in a clinical trial setting.

Lifestyle modifications

Avoidance of trigger factors

One of the most common trigger factors for atopic eczema is the house-dust mite, as indicated by strong circumstantial evidence. For example, cutaneous skin patch tests with house-dust mite extract produce an eczematous reaction involving allergen-specific helper T lymphocytes in patients with atopic eczema.[5] Reducing the level of house-dust mites in the living environment, by methods such as frequent vacuum cleaning, use of acaricidal sprays and the use of mattress and pillow covers which are impervious to mites, is often advised as a strategy to improve the symptoms of atopic eczema as well as other atopic conditions such as allergic rhinitis and asthma.[5] Killing the mites is not effective unless the allergenic dead mites and their faeces are also removed.

Randomised controlled trials examining the effects of removing house-dust mites on established atopic eczema have supported the use of intensive dust mite eradication regimens, particularly vacuum cleaning. These strategies are also effective in reducing levels of animal dander, which is also a common trigger factor for atopic eczema. However, in order to induce detectable benefits, there must be an extreme reduction in house-dust mite populations, and the measures required for only a modest symptomatic benefit may be impractical for many people.[14] Aside from this demand on time, this approach may also incur significant costs for a high-filtration vacuum cleaner, impermeable mattress covers and mite sprays.[5]

> Randomised controlled trials examining the effects of removing house-dust mites on established atopic eczema have supported the use of intensive dust mite eradication regimens.

In addition to the use of impermeable mattress and pillow covers, bedding and clothing may be selected on the basis of its texture or fabric composition. Cottons are fine-textured and breathe well, and are considered a good choice for patients with atopic eczema, though the texture, rather than the actual choice of fabric, is probably the most important factor.[5,14] Although sensitisation to lanolin remains relatively uncommon, the texture of woollen products may irritate existing eczematous areas.[41]

Due to their
destructive effect
on the skin's
protective lipid
barrier, soaps and
detergents can
induce skin
dryness and
itchiness in
patients with
atopic eczema.

Due to their destructive effect on the skin's protective lipid barrier, soaps and detergents can induce skin dryness and itchiness in patients with atopic eczema. Use of bubble bath and shampoos in the bath should therefore be avoided, and emollient soap substitutes should be encouraged.[14] Similarly, use of non-biological washing powders and avoidance of fabric conditioners may act to reduce levels of irritation to the skin.[42] Furthermore, many toiletries contain perfumes, preservatives and alcohols which may prove irritating to eczematous skin.[14]

Although food hypersensitivity is frequently blamed for eczema exacerbations, diet is only reported to be a significant trigger factor in approximately 10% of children, and considerably less so in adults.[14] Dietary modification is generally only recommended for patients whose eczema is uncontrolled by conventional treatment options. If food hypersensitivity is a trigger for exacerbations of eczema, it may manifest as increased itchiness immediately after eating certain foods, and hence be relatively easy to identify. It may also induce symptoms such as skin swelling and redness, abdominal pain, vomiting, wheezing, itchy eyes and sneezing, as long as 24 hours after ingestion. An 'exclusion-and-challenge' procedure, overseen by a dietitian, can confirm a food hypersensitivity diagnosis. The most common trigger foods include cow's milk, eggs, soya, wheat, fish and peanuts.[14] Elimination diets are difficult for patients and their families to adhere to, even within a clinical trial setting.[5]

Skin care

Various aspects of good skin care have been discussed elsewhere in this section. The use of emollients to normalise the hydration of the skin is strongly recommended, as is the avoidance of exposure to soaps and detergents wherever possible.[5,14] It is advised that emollients be applied generously at least three times a day, and as soon as possible after bathing or showering, whilst water is still trapped in the skin.[14] The use of salt baths is a further option, due to its weak antiseptic properties, and its ability to draw fluid out of oedematous acute eczematous skin. However, controlled trial data assessing the value of salt baths is sparse. This strategy is based mainly on anecdotal evidence, not least arising from reports of the effectiveness of the combination of sea salt and UV light exposure for visitors to the Dead Sea.[5]

Reducing scratching

Particularly in children, who do not appreciate the dangers of the 'itch–scratch cycle', it is important to take measures to try and minimise scratching. In addition to reducing the exposure to allergens, as described above, children's nails should be kept short, cotton mittens may be worn at night, and distraction is often most effective during the day.[42]

Psychological approaches

It is recognised that psychological stress is an important factor in provoking, exacerbating and prolonging atopic eczema, though the mechanistic link remains unclear.[43] The prevailing view focuses on stress-induced release of hormones and neuropeptides into the circulation, and their subsequent regulation of immune and neurogenic inflammatory reactions.[44] Furthermore, it is becoming apparent that psychological stress can directly impair skin barrier function. There is evidence to suggest that this is a result of reduced epidermal lipid synthesis (cholesterol, fatty acids and ceramide).[43]

Although psychological stress appears to contribute to the worsening of atopic eczema, it is also a manifestation of the condition. Atopic eczema is associated with a considerable impairment of health-related quality of life, particularly due to itchiness, which can be particularly distressing in children.[45,46] There is likely to be a considerable psychological component involved in the 'itch–scratch' cycle. The value of stress reduction techniques, such as group psychotherapy, has been assessed in clinical trials, with long-term reductions in corticosteroid use reported.[47,48] In addition to relaxation techniques, behavioural modifications aimed at reducing the exacerbation of symptoms caused by scratching may be beneficial. Patient education about the nature of the disease and its treatment is also advantageous. For example, education of parents of children with atopic eczema has been shown to improve compliance to treatment regimens.[49]

> The value of stress reduction techniques, such as group psychotherapy, has been assessed in clinical trials, with long-term reductions in corticosteroid use reported.

Breast-feeding

Although not strictly a management option, breastfeeding is a lifestyle feature which warrants discussion here, due to the debate over whether it is protective or harmful in the context of altering the risk of atopic eczema in the infant. Breastfeeding has long been considered to be protective against atopic diseases, and this is not without scientific justification. The presence of immunoglobulin antibodies in human milk, for example, may prevent antigen absorption and the subsequent triggering of immunoglobulin E (IgE) production.[50] However, human breast milk contains proteins which are foreign to the infant, and specific IgE to human milk proteins has been detected in the sera of atopic infants.[51] Accordingly, there is some trial data to indicate that breast-feeding is not protective, and may even be a risk factor for atopy, in some infants.[50] Trials are subject to considerable ethical constraints, however (e.g. randomisation to breast-feeding is not possible), and are confounded by numerous factors, such as genetic predisposition and non-exclusive use of breast/cow's milk.[52]

Thus, there does appear to be a subgroup of patients who may not benefit from breast-feeding in terms of the risk of developing atopic eczema.[50] However, given that this population is yet to be defined, and considering the numerous other advantages of breast-feeding, it continues to be advocated in international guidelines, at least for the first 4–6 months after birth.[53]

Key points

- The management of atopic eczema involves a wide range of treatment options and lifestyle modifications. The evidence base supporting the efficacy and safety of these approaches varies considerably.

- Topical corticosteroids are the first-line option for treatment of eczema exacerbations. Despite a lack of abundant clinical data, their use is well established, and safety concerns are, to a large extent, unjustified if dosing guidelines are adhered to.

- Emollients and moisturisers are widely used as a prophylactic therapy. There is strong scientific rationale for their use, though clinical data in support of their efficacy are extremely sparse.

- The most recent development in treatment options is the emergence of two topically administered immunosuppressant drugs, which may be used if a patient's symptoms are uncontrolled using more conventional topical corticosteroid drugs.

- The benefits of antihistamines for atopic eczema lie mainly in their central, sedative effects, rather than their antipruritic properties.

- Antibiotics may be used in cases of secondary infection, often in combination with topical corticosteroids. Probiotics, in contrast, may prove beneficial in reducing eczema severity in infants.

- Phototherapy is a long-established treatment strategy for dermatological disorders, though there are considerable and insufficiently addressed long-term safety concerns.

- Traditional Chinese medicine has demonstrated some benefits outside of controlled clinical trials, though these may be due to the unregulated content of steroids and other drugs, which helps to explain the dubious safety profile.

- Homeopathy and dietary supplements are used by many patients, but no significant efficacy has been demonstrated in a trial setting.

- Lifestyle modifications, including allergen avoidance, skin care and psychological approaches, impose demands on the time and resources of patients, but are associated with some proven benefits.

References

A list of the published evidence which has been reviewed in compiling the preceding section of *BESTMEDICINE*.

1 Ellis C, Luger T, Abeck D *et al.* International Consensus Conference on Atopic Dermatitis II (ICCAD II): clinical update and current treatment strategies. *Br J Dermatol* 2003; **148(Suppl 63)**: 3–10.

2 Guidelines for the management of atopic eczema – Primary Care Dermatology Society and British Association of Dermatologists. *www.bad.org.uk*

3 Topical steroids for atopic dermatitis in primary care. *Drug Ther Bull* 2003; **41**: 5–8.

4 *British National Formulary (BNF) 49.* London: the British Medical Association and the Royal Pharmaceutical Society of Great Britain. March, 2005.

5 Hoare C, Li Wan Po A, Williams H. Systematic review of treatments for atopic eczema. *Health Technol Assess* 2000; **4**: 1–191.

6 Kragballe K. Topical corticosteroids: mechanisms of action. *Acta Derm Venereol Suppl (Stockh)* 1989; **151**: 7–10.

7 Barnes PJ. Anti-inflammatory actions of glucocorticoids: molecular mechanisms. *Clin Sci (Lond)* 1998; **94**: 557–72.

8 Leung DY. Infection in atopic dermatitis. *Curr Opin Pediatr* 2003; **15**: 399–404.

9 Wachs GN, Maibach HI. Co-operative double-blind trial of an antibiotic/corticoid combination in impetiginized atopic dermatitis. *Br J Dermatol* 1976; **95**: 323–8.

10 Hjorth N, Schmidt H, Thomsen K. Fusidic acid plus betamethasone in infected or potentially infected eczema. *Pharmatherapeutica* 1985; **4**: 126–31.

11 Ramsay CA, Savoie JM, Gilbert M, Gidon M, Kidson P. The treatment of atopic dermatitis with topical fusidic acid and hydrocortisone acetate. *J Euro Acad Derm Ven* 1996; **7**: S15–S22.

12 Furue M, Terao H, Rikihisa W *et al.* Clinical dose and adverse effects of topical steroids in daily management of atopic dermatitis. *Br J Dermatol* 2003; **148**: 128–33.

13 National Institute for Clinical Excellence (NICE). Final Appraisal Determination. Frequency of application of topical corticosteroids for atopic eczema. April 2004. *www.nice.org.uk*

14 Prodigy Guidance – Atopic eczema. *www.prodigy.nhs.uk.*

15 Lagos BR, Maibach HI. Frequency of application of topical corticosteroids: an overview. *Br J Dermatol* 1998; **139**: 763–6.

16 Loden M. The skin barrier and use of moisturizers in atopic dermatitis. *Clin Dermatol* 2003; **21**: 145–57.

17 Billmann-Eberwein C, Rippke F, Ruzicka T, Krutmann J. Modulation of atopy patch test reactions by topical treatment of human skin with a fatty acid-rich emollient. *Skin Pharmacol Appl Skin Physiol* 2002; **15**: 100–4.

18 Hanifin J, Hebert AA, Mays SR *et al.* Effects of a low-potency corticosteroid lotion plus a moisturizing regimen in the treatment of atopic dermatitis. *Curr Ther Res Clin Exp* 1998; **59**: 227–33.

19 Wilhelm KP, Schloermann A. Efficacy and tolerability of a topical preparation containing 10% urea in patients with atopic dermatitis. *Aktuel Dermatol* 1998; **24**: 26–30.

20 Larregue M, Devaux J, Audebert C, Gelmetti DR. A double-blind controlled study on the efficacy and tolerability of 6% ammonium lactate cream in children with atopic dermatitis. *Nouv Dermatol* 1996; **15**: 720–1.

21 Lack G, Fox D, Northstone K, Golding J. Factors associated with the development of peanut allergy in childhood. *N Engl J Med* 2003; **348**: 977–85.

22 Khandpur S, Sharma VK, Sumanth K. Topical immunomodulators in dermatology. *J Postgrad Med* 2004; **50**: 131–9.

23 Reitamo S, Rustin M, Ruzicka T *et al.* Efficacy and safety of tacrolimus ointment compared with that of hydrocortisone butyrate ointment in adult patients with atopic dermatitis. *J Allergy Clin Immunol* 2002; **109**: 547–55.

24 Reitamo S, Van Leent EJ, Ho V *et al.* Efficacy and safety of tacrolimus ointment compared with that of hydrocortisone acetate ointment in children with atopic dermatitis. *J Allergy Clin Immunol* 2002; **109**: 539–46.

25 Eichenfield LF, Lucky AW, Boguniewicz M *et al.* Safety and efficacy of pimecrolimus (ASM 981) cream 1% in the treatment of mild and moderate atopic dermatitis in children and adolescents. *J Am Acad Dermatol* 2002; **46**: 495–504.

26 La Rosa M, Ranno C, Musarra I *et al.* Double-blind study of cetirizine in atopic eczema in children. *Ann Allergy* 1994; **73**: 117–22.

27 Munday J, Bloomfield R, Goldman M *et al.* Chlorpheniramine is no more effective than placebo in relieving the symptoms of childhood atopic dermatitis with a nocturnal itching and scratching component. *Dermatology* 2002; **205**: 40–5.

28 Wollenberg A, Wetzel S, Burgdorf WH, Haas J. Viral infections in atopic dermatitis: pathogenic aspects and clinical management. *J Allergy Clin Immunol* 2003; **112**: 667–74.

29 Isolauri E, Arvola T, Sutas Y, Moilanen E, Salminen S. Probiotics in the management of atopic eczema. *Clin Exp Allergy* 2000; **30**: 1604–10.

30 Sowden JM, Berth-Jones J, Ross JS *et al.* Double-blind, controlled, crossover study of cyclosporin in adults with severe refractory atopic dermatitis. *Lancet* 1991; **338**: 137–40.

31 Scheinfeld NS, Tutrone WD, Weinberg JM, DeLeo VA. Phototherapy of atopic dermatitis. *Clin Dermatol* 2003; **21**: 241–8.

32 Krutmann J, Medve-Koenigs K, Ruzicka T, Ranft U, Wilkens JH. Ultraviolet-free phototherapy. *Photodermatol Photoimmunol Photomed* 2005; **21**: 59–61.

33 Goodyear HM, Harper JI. 'Wet wrap' dressings for eczema: an effective treatment but not to be misused. *Br J Dermatol* 2002; **146**: 159.

34 Zhang W, Leonard T, Bath-Hextall F *et al.* Chinese herbal medicine for atopic eczema. *Cochrane Database Syst Rev* 2004: CD002291.

35 Artik S, Ruzicka T. Complementary therapy for atopic eczema and other allergic skin diseases. *Dermatol Ther* 2003; **16**: 150–63.

36 NHS Direct – Acupuncture. *www.nhsdirect.nhs.uk*

37 Chen CJ, Yu HS. Acupuncture, electrostimulation, and reflex therapy in dermatology. *Dermatol Ther* 2003; **16**: 87–92.

38 Smolle J. Homeopathy in dermatology. *Dermatol Ther* 2003; **16**: 93–7.

39 Schachner L, Field T, Hernandez-Reif M, Duarte AM, Krasnegor J. Atopic dermatitis symptoms decreased in children following massage therapy. *Pediatr Dermatol* 1998; **15**: 390–5.

40 Anderson C, Lis-Balchin M, Kirk-Smith M. Evaluation of massage with essential oils on childhood atopic eczema. *Phytother Res* 2000; **14**: 452–6.

41 Wakelin SH, Smith H, White IR, Rycroft RJ, McFadden JP. A retrospective analysis of contact allergy to lanolin. *Br J Dermatol* 2001; **145**: 28–31.

42 National Eczema Society. *www.eczema.org*

43 Choi EH, Brown BE, Crumrine D *et al.* Mechanisms by which psychologic stress alters cutaneous permeability barrier homeostasis and stratum corneum integrity. *J Invest Dermatol* 2005; **124**: 587–95.

44 Wright RJ, Cohen RT, Cohen S. The impact of stress on the development and expression of atopy. *Curr Opin Allergy Clin Immunol* 2005; **5**: 23–9.

45 Kiebert G, Sorensen SV, Revicki D *et al.* Atopic dermatitis is associated with a decrement in health-related quality of life. *Int J Dermatol* 2002; **41**: 151–8.

46 Ben-Gashir MA, Seed PT, Hay RJ. Quality of life and disease severity are correlated in children with atopic dermatitis. *Br J Dermatol* 2004; **150**: 284–90.

47 Cole WC, Roth HL, Sachs LB. Group psychotherapy as an aid in the medical treatment of eczema. *J Am Acad Dermatol* 1988; **18**: 286–91.

48 Horne DJ, White AE, Varigos GA. A preliminary study of psychological therapy in the management of atopic eczema. *Br J Med Psychol* 1989; **62(Pt 3)**: 241–8.

49 Broberg A, Kalimo K, Lindblad B, Swanbeck G. Parental education in the treatment of childhood atopic eczema. *Acta Derm Venereol* 1990; **70**: 495–9.

50 Eigenmann PA. Breast-feeding and atopic eczema dermatitis syndrome: protective or harmful? *Allergy* 2004; **59(Suppl 78)**: 42–4.

51 Cantisani A, Giuffrida MG, Fabris C *et al.* Detection of specific IgE to human milk proteins in sera of atopic infants. *FEBS Lett* 1997; **412**: 515–7.

52 Bergmann RL, Diepgen TL, Kuss O *et al.* Breastfeeding duration is a risk factor for atopic eczema. *Clin Exp Allergy* 2002; **32**: 205–9.

53 Host A, Koletzko B, Dreborg S *et al.* Dietary products used in infants for treatment and prevention of food allergy. Joint Statement of the European Society for Paediatric Allergology and Clinical Immunology (ESPACI) Committee on Hypoallergenic Formulas and the European Society for Paediatric Gastroenterology, Hepatology and Nutrition (ESPGHAN) Committee on Nutrition. *Arch Dis Child* 1999; **81**: 80–4.

Acknowledgements

Figure 1 is adapted from Barnes, 1998.[7]
Figure 2 is adapted from Loden, 2003.[16]

PATIENT NOTES
Dr Tim Mitchell

The skin – a multifunctional organ

Most people probably do not think of the skin as anything other than an outer layer of the body, but it is really another organ. Just like the liver or the kidneys, the skin carries out several different and very important functions. Although the skin seems very thin, it is in fact the largest organ in the body with a surface area of 1.8 m^2 and comprising about 16% of our total body weight.

Before looking at the causes and impact of skin diseases such as eczema, it is worth considering some of the more important functions of the skin.

- A barrier to physical agents, including UV radiation.
- Protection from mechanical injury.
- Defence against invading microbes.
- Homeostasis (the prevention of loss of water and electrolytes).
- Regulation of temperature and insulation.
- Sensory functions.
- Fine touch and grip.
- Vitamin D synthesis.
- A calorie store (in the subcutaneous fat that is present).
- Cosmetic, psychosocial and display functions.

Any disease that affects even a few of these functions is likely to have a major effect on the functioning of the whole person, both physically and psychologically.

Eczema – types and terminology

Eczema is one of these skin diseases, and can have a variety of different causes and names. Atopic eczema (the main subject of this book) is probably the best known, but there is also contact eczema (which can be irritant or allergic), discoid eczema, seborrhoeic eczema and eczema associated with poor circulation in the legs and varicose veins (also referred to as varicose, stasis or gravitational eczema).

Atopic eczema (or atopic dermatitis as it is sometimes referred to) is the most common chronic skin disease in childhood and although the majority of cases clear up before the patient enters adulthood, the affected individual remains vulnerable to recurrences (exacerbations) of the condition. Cases that persist and continue to recur appear to have an important element of irritation from, or allergy to, a variety of substances that regularly come into contact with the skin. Contact eczema is much more common in adults than in children, and is often caused by

Atopic eczema is the most common chronic skin disease in childhood.

People who are 'atopic' have a tendency to suffer from eczema, asthma and hay fever – the so-called atopic triad.

contact with substances that an individual is exposed to in their place of work.

This edition of *BESTMEDICINE* focuses on atopic eczema because it is the most common type of eczema, much of the research into eczema and its treatments are based upon it, and the basic problem in the skin is much the same as it is for the other types. As will be shown later, the principles of treatment for the different types are also similar.

The word 'atopic' comes from the term 'atopy', which refers to an abnormal triggering of immune proteins in the body in response to 'trigger' substances in the environment. People who are 'atopic' have a tendency to suffer from eczema, asthma and hay fever – the so-called atopic triad. In hay fever, the environmental trigger is pollen, whilst in asthma and eczema the triggers are not as clearly identified.

There can be some confusion over the difference between the words 'eczema' and 'dermatitis'. Eczema comes from the Greek word for 'boiling' – a good description of how the skin can feel in acute eczema. Dermatitis really means 'inflammation of the skin' and can be used to describe other forms of disease that cause inflammation. The use of the word 'dermatitis' was often taken to mean that the skin problem was caused by an external factor and, if the person was in work, some form of compensation might be involved. Some forms of eczema are often referred to as dermatitis – for example, seborrhoeic dermatitis and when the napkin area is affected – but for simplicity it is better to stick to the use of eczema to avoid confusion.

The burden of eczema in the UK

Eczema is a very common problem. In the UK, skin problems account for somewhere between 15 and 20% of all consultations in general practice, whilst eczema accounts for 30% of these cases. Therefore, about 5% of all patients seeing a GP will be seeking advice for eczema. In hospital dermatology departments, where many of the less common conditions are concentrated, eczema accounts for 14% of the total dermatological workload.

Why does eczema occur?

The Disease Overview section earlier in this book discusses the changes that occur within the skin. For simplicity, these changes can be looked at as a failing brick wall. The skin cells near the surface are lined up much like bricks in a wall with overlapping layers stacked on one another. The 'mortar' holding the wall together is a substance rich in lipids (types of fats), which provides extra waterproofing and adds to the important physical barrier functions that have been described previously. The skin acts as a barrier to substances getting in, as well as heat and fluid getting out. However, this barrier starts to fail when fluid collects in the outer layers of the skin, which then forces the skin cells apart. This causes the outer layer to resemble a sponge, hence the term spongiosis used by doctors; it also leaks like one! The small blood vessels supplying the skin become wider and supply more blood than usual, leading to the redness and heat that is common in acute eczema. If the eczema is not treated and it becomes chronic, spongiosis is not seen and the outer layer of the skin becomes thickened and rough. The blood vessels are still wider than normal but the increased thickness of the skin stops it looking so hot and red. Chronic scratching can also encourage this thickening leading to areas of skin with increased skin markings (fine creases) – a process called lichenification. The whole process in eczema can become complicated leading to different presentations of the disease.

Complications of eczema

Bacterial infections

The breakdown of the barrier function of the skin can let infection in. This is especially common in atopic eczema, where rough or broken skin leads to a much higher level of colonisation by bacteria – most commonly by *Staphylococcus*. The infected areas will look different from the rest of the affected skin, with more redness and pain, the appearance of green or yellow spots of pus ('pustules') and/or large blisters with clear or milky contents (impetigo). If the bacteria get in beyond the skin there can also be a general (systemic) upset with a raised temperature. If the infection is due to *Staphylococcus*, there can be additional problems as these bacteria produce a toxin that results in a type of allergic reaction. This triggers a vicious cycle in which the immune system releases substances which produce more inflammation, leading to a worsening of the eczema and providing greater opportunities for infection.

Herpes simplex infection

In the atopic person, the cold sore virus, herpes simplex, can produce a much more widespread outbreak of grouped vesicles (very small blisters), which break down to produce little erosions. In a baby this can be a very serious infection (called eczema herpeticum) and requires urgent antiviral treatment through a drip or injections in hospital.

Allergic reaction to treatment

If eczema gets worse rather than better with treatment, this could be because an allergy has developed to one or more of the ingredients in the cream or ointment. This is especially likely to occur with eczema on the lower legs (varicose eczema). The allergy can be due to active materials such as hydrocortisone,

The whole process in eczema can become complicated leading to different presentations of the disease.

antiseptics or antibiotics, and also to chemicals in the base of the cream or ointment such as the preservative.

Erythroderma and exfoliative dermatitis

With some kinds of eczema the skin can become red all over and is often scaly as well. This situation is called erythroderma if the redness predominates, or exfoliative dermatitis if there is prominent scaling. When the entire skin is affected, various problems can occur: normal temperature regulation can be lost, excessive fluid is lost through the skin, there is strain on the heart and, if untreated, heart failure may occur. This is another situation in which hospital admission is necessary.

Diagnosing eczema

Many patients expect to have investigations carried out to prove the diagnosis but, as we have seen in the Disease Overview, there are no specific tests for eczema and the diagnosis is made principally on the basis of a personal and family history of the condition, and on the findings of a skin examination.

Some additional investigations may help to clarify these findings, depending on the certainty of the diagnosis of eczema, what type of eczema it is and whether there are any suspected complications. For example, swabs and other skin tests can be taken to look for signs of infection, and specialised skin allergy tests can be carried out to determine the cause of the exacerbation. These latter investigations are called patch tests and are usually only carried out in hospital.

Although many patients suspect food allergy as the root of their eczema, in truth it is not a very common cause. Such allergies may only be a problem in about 6% of infants with an early onset of atopic eczema, and are far less common for adults. Food allergies causing eczema can be very difficult to diagnose but blood tests can be taken to look at reactions to specific foods. These are called RAST tests, which stands for radioallergosorbent. The involvement of a dietitian and/or an immunologist can help to determine the cause of the food allergy. However, there is no single general test that will point towards an allergic cause. As with many allergies, a correct diagnosis requires the demonstration of benefit from withdrawing the suspected food, relapse when it is reinstated in the diet, and remission when it is again withdrawn.

Clinical management of atopic eczema – general principles

The following sections of this book will deal in detail with the evidence underlying the use of the two most recently introduced

> *Diagnosis is made principally on the basis of a personal and family history of the condition.*

treatments for atopic eczema, but it is worth looking at the general principles underpinning the treatment of the condition. It may be better to use the word 'management' as ensuring the eczema gets better often involves much more than just creams and ointments. The essentials of good clinical management of eczema are outlined below.

- Establish what anxieties and questions the patient or their family may have.
- Identify the impact that the eczema has on the patient's quality of life (e.g. loss of sleep, absence from school or work etc.)
- Explore what makes the eczema worse; these questions can sometimes lead to useful tests and often point to measures that will help protect the skin (e.g. using a greasy ointment when in the swimming pool). By identifying these factors, the individual can make efforts to avoid exposing themselves to them, wherever this is possible.
- For the dryness of the skin associated with eczema it may be necessary to use emollients. These can be in the form of creams, ointments and oils dispersed in the bath. Relieving the dryness may also help the itch that is commonplace with eczema. The best emollient for any patient is the one that feels best. This may require trying a few different types whilst several different ones may be needed for different parts of the body. Emollients based on grease alone (e.g. soft white paraffin and emulsifying ointment) are often very well tolerated (i.e. they do not sting or irritate), but are less attractive cosmetically. Emollients should be applied as often as needed, and are prescribed or bought in large quantities such as 500 gram tubs.
- Soap substitutes (consisting of dispersible oils) are available for use in the bath or shower, which not only help to make the skin less dry but also cleanse it. Avoiding soap prevents further damage to the 'mortar in the brick wall' as the lipids in between the cells are damaged by detergents.
- Where any infection occurs it should be treated promptly. Failure to do so is a common reason for eczema deteriorating. The use of a suitable antibiotic should clear up most infections.
- Most cases of eczema will improve by applying a suitable topical steroid. This should be sufficiently potent to produce real benefit but should not be used for longer than necessary.

By following these simple guidelines, most people's eczema can be brought under control and kept from flaring up too often with care from their GP. However, sometimes help is needed from a dermatologist. To help GPs decide when it is necessary to refer a particular patient to a dermatologist, the National Institute for Clinical Excellence (NICE) has produced guidelines for a number of different skin diseases. One of these guidelines is

Ensuring the eczema gets better often involves much more than just creams and ointments.

for the management of children with atopic eczema. In this document it is accepted that "most children with atopic eczema can be managed in primary care" but then lists reasons for referral to a specialist service including:

- suspected severe infection with herpes simplex (eczema herpeticum)
- the disease is severe and has not responded to appropriate therapy
- the rash becomes infected with bacteria, and treatment with an oral antibiotic plus a topical corticosteroid has failed
- treatment requires the use of excessive amounts of potent topical corticosteroids
- management has not controlled the rash satisfactorily (ultimately, failure to improve is probably best based on a subjective assessment by the child or parent)
- the patient or their family may benefit from additional advice on different methods of applying treatment (e.g. bandaging techniques)
- contact dermatitis is suspected and its confirmation requires patch testing
- dietary factors are suspected and dietary control is a possibility
- the diagnosis is, or has, become uncertain.

Other approaches to eczema management

Some patients can become very stressed by the symptoms and appearance of chronic eczema, and specialists other than dermatologists can be very helpful in dealing with this stress. Cognitive behavioural therapy (CBT) is a psychological approach that examines thought processes. When it comes to eczema CBT can help by modifying:

- inaccurate and unhelpful beliefs
- ineffective coping behaviour
- negative mood states.

This approach can therefore alleviate anxiety and help patients to move towards having a sense of control over their eczema. The doctor needs to ensure that this sense of control is realistic and based on a good understanding of the disease and the benefits (and indeed the limitations) of treatment.

Some patients may also wish to consult a complementary practitioner for alternative approaches to treatment. The patient then moves away from an evidence-based approach to a 'belief-based' approach, as it is very difficult to carry out research on alternative treatments. However, it does appear that homeopathy, acupuncture and hypnotherapy can be beneficial in some patients in improving the eczema itself, reducing the associated stress and controlling the sense of itch.

Cognitive behavioural therapy can alleviate anxiety and help patients to move towards having a sense of control over their eczema.

3. Drug review – Pimecrolimus (Elidel®)

Dr Scott Chambers and Dr Eleanor Bull
CSF Medical Communications Ltd

Summary

Topical corticosteroids are recognised along with emollients as first-line treatment options for atopic eczema. However, prolonged use of corticosteroids can be associated with significant local and systemic side-effects, in addition to tachyphylaxis and symptom rebound after withdrawal. The availability of a new non-steroidal calcineurin inhibitor, pimecrolimus, offers the promise of good efficacy in the treatment of atopic eczema without many of the detrimental side-effects of corticosteroids. Pimecrolimus acts by inhibiting cytokine expression from activated T cells – a central factor in the development of atopic eczema. As a consequence of its novel chemical structure, pimecrolimus is not absorbed systemically to any great extent, thereby minimising the likelihood of adverse systemic immune effects. Thus, pimecrolimus has skin-selective anti-inflammatory effects, and unlike corticosteroids, has no skin atrophogenic potential. In clinical terms, a large-scale clinical trials programme has demonstrated its effectiveness in both the short-term treatment of atopic eczema and in preventing the progression of disease flares in adults and children over 2 years of age. Pimecrolimus is well tolerated, with the principal adverse event being a transient mild-to-moderate application site irritation.

Introduction

The established first-line treatment option for atopic eczema has for some time been the use of emollients and topical corticosteroids. However, there has been significant concern relating to prolonged use of topical corticosteroids, principally due to symptom rebound after treatment withdrawal, local side-effects, systemic adverse effects and tachyphylaxis. Local adverse reactions reported to occur include skin atrophy, telangiectasia and hypopigmentation. In addition, systemic absorption of corticosteroids can be associated with other more serious adverse effects, including suppression of the hypothalamic–pituitary–

There is a
clinical need for
alternative agents
which offer
effective
management of
atopic eczema
without such
detrimental
side-effects.

adrenal axis, growth retardation and Cushing's syndrome. Consequently, these adverse effects have engendered a degree of mistrust of corticosteroids amongst some physicians and the wider population – a phenomenon which has been coined steroid phobia[1] – with the potential for subsequent treatment non-adherence. Thus, there is a clinical need for alternative agents which offer effective management of atopic eczema without such detrimental side-effects.

Pimecrolimus is a novel non-steroidal anti-inflammatory and immunomodulatory agent, specifically developed for the treatment of inflammatory skin disorders, which is licensed for the treatment of atopic eczema. It is a macrolide-related agent derived from asomycin, and selectively acts upon T lymphocytes and mast cells in the skin leading to inhibition of the production and release of cytokines and other inflammatory mediators. Of note is the fact that unlike corticosteroids, pimecrolimus does not cause skin atrophy thereby allowing it to be used in sensitive areas of the body, including the face. Pimecrolimus is a cell-specific inhibitor of cytokines and thus selectively targets inflammation in the skin without leading to any impairment of the systemic immune response. This contrasts to other agents used in the management of the condition including tacrolimus, ciclosporin and the corticosteroids.

Pimecrolimus is licensed in the UK for the short-term treatment of mild-to-moderate eczema, and for intermittent long-term prevention of progression to disease flares. However, pimecrolimus is not currently recommended for use in children under 2 years of age. Consequently, whilst the clinical trial programme has specifically examined this infant patient population together with its potential in other inflammatory dermatological conditions, data reviewed in this edition of *BESTMEDICINE* will reflect only those data which supports the use of pimecrolimus within its UK license.

Pharmacology and pharmacokinetics
Chemistry

The chemistry of
pimecrolimus is of
essentially academic
interest and most
healthcare
professionals will, like
you, skip this section.

Pimecrolimus is a natural derivative of the macrolactam asomycin developed from *Streptomyces hygroscopicus var. ascomyceticus*. The chemical structure of pimecrolimus is shown in Figure 1. Whilst pimecrolimus is chemically related to tacrolimus – another macrolactam derivative licensed for use in atopic eczema – pimecrolimus has a number of distinct structural differences which confer significantly greater lipophilicity and translate into a distinct pharmacological profile.

Mode of action and pharmacodynamics

The mechanism of action of pimecrolimus has yet to be fully elucidated. However, it is believed to act in a similar manner to tacrolimus and

Figure 1. Chemical structure of pimecrolimus.

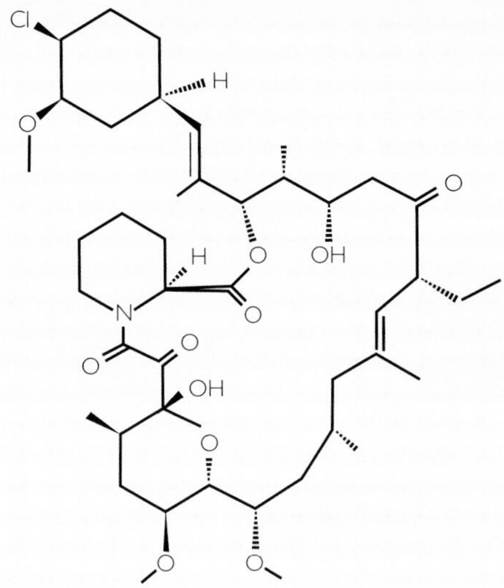

ciclosporin by binding with a high affinity (IC_{50}=1.8 nmol/L) to a cytosolic T-cell receptor called macrophillin-12 (FKBP-12).[2,3] This results in the inhibition of a calcium-dependent protein phosphatase – calcineurin – a key-signalling mediator involved in the transcriptional activation of various early acting cytokines. Thus, binding of pimecrolimus to macrophillin-12 prevents calcineurin-mediated dephosphorylation of the nuclear factor of activated T cells (NF-AT), which prevents its translocation into the nucleus and subsequent binding to its nuclear-localised binding partner, a normal response in T-cell activation (Figure 2). This prevents the formation of an active transcription factor complex involved in the expression of both Th1 (interleukin [IL]-2 and inteferon γ)- and Th2 (IL-4 and IL-10)-type cytokines in activated T cells. The production of other cytokines such as IL-5 and tumour necrosis factor (TNF)-α is also down-regulated by pimecrolimus, whilst pimecrolimus also inhibits the antigen–immunoglobulin (Ig)E stimulated activation of mast cells, thereby preventing the release of various pre-formed inflammatory mediators such as histamine, hexosaminidase and tryptase.[4,5] Pimecrolimus is highly selective for T cells, with no effect on the proliferation of keratinocytes, fibroblasts or endothelial cells. It also down-regulates coreceptors which are necessary for the activation and expansion of inflammatory effector T cells, thereby further potentiating its potent T-cell selective activity.[6] In contrast to corticosteroids, pimecrolimus has no effect on Langerhans cells, which are key immune cells involved in local skin immunosurveillance.[7]

> Pimecrolimus prevents the formation of an active transcription factor complex involved in the expression of both Th1 and Th2 type cytokines in activated T cells.

Figure 2. Pimecrolimus blocks expression of cytokines from activated T cells: a proposed mechanism of action.
IL, interleukin; NF–AT, nuclear factor of activated T cells.

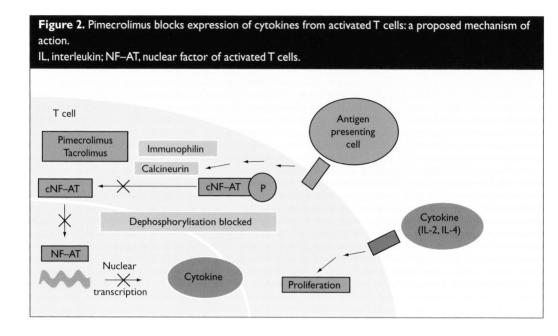

Pharmacokinetics

☛ *The pharmacokinetics of a drug are of interest to healthcare professionals because it is important for them to understand the action of a drug on the body over a period of time.*

In a non-controlled, open-labelled study of 12 adult patients with moderate-to-severe atopic eczema, treated twice daily with pimecrolimus, 1%, for 3 weeks, blood concentrations of the agent remained very low.[8] In 78% of samples evaluated, the concentrations of pimecrolimus remained below the level of quantification (0.5 ng/mL), whilst the highest concentration reported was 1.4 ng/mL. Thus, pimecrolimus does not appear to be extensively absorbed after repeated application. Furthermore, there was no evidence of significant drug accumulation with longer periods of treatment. Amongst patients with the largest affected areas of eczema, consistently low blood levels of pimecrolimus were reported. Thus, pimecrolimus has low bioavailablity and therefore, minimal potential for suppressing systemic immune responses. This factor is of particular importance when applying topical agents to paediatric patients, who have a lower body surface area to mass ratio.

A preliminary pharmacokinetic study in paediatric patients (n=10) with moderate-to-severe atopic eczema, examined the systemic absorption of pimecrolimus, 1%, applied twice daily for 3 weeks.[9] Patients had up to 69% of their body surface area affected (BSA) and thus significant areas of the body were exposed to active treatment. Despite this, consistently low blood concentrations of pimecrolimus were reported in this study with the majority of blood samples being below the limit of quantification (0.5 ng/mL). This was supported by further open-label, non-controlled, multiple-dose studies in paediatric and infant patient populations with extensive atopic dermatitis.[10] Again, consistently low blood concentrations of pimecrolimus were reported, indicating minimal systemic exposure.

Due to the low systemic bioavailability of pimecrolimus, assessment of standard pharmacokinetic parameters is problematic, and therefore these can be determined only when using oral formulations of pimecrolimus. As such, the clinical relevance of such parameters is questionable. However, a single radiolabelled oral dose of pimecrolimus undergoes metabolism via cytochrome (CYP) 3A4, and is excreted principally via faeces as metabolites, with only a small fraction eliminated in urine.[11]

Preclinical pharmacology

A number of animal models of inflammatory dermatological disorders have evaluated the efficacy of topical and oral formulations of pimecrolimus, and have demonstrated its potent and skin-selective immunosuppressive effects together with its minimal side-effects on the systemic immune response.

In a porcine model of allergic contact dermatitis, pimecrolimus was shown to be at least as effective as highly potent corticosteroids.[12] Significant anti-inflammatory effects were observed with concentrations as low as 0.04%. Furthermore, no skin atrophogenic potential was observed with pimecrolimus, in contrast with the corticosteroids which were shown to cause skin atrophy and altered skin texture in these animals.[13] Pigs are particularly good models for skin inflammatory disorders, given the similarity in permeability and general structure of its skin with human skin.

When oral formulations of pimecrolimus, tacrolimus and ciclosporin were administered in mice and rat models of allergic contact dermatitis, pimecrolimus was shown to be highly effective in reducing inflammation.[12] Moreover, in the rat model, oral pimecrolimus was shown to be more effective in reducing the signs of allergic contact dermatitis than ciclosporin.

In hypomagnesaemic hairless rats (a model of atopic eczema in which a transient erythematous rash develops with generalised pruritus), topical and oral pimecrolimus were shown to reduce skin inflammation and pruritus selectively and effectively.[14] In addition, both formulations of pimecrolimus were shown to have prophylactic activity.

In addition to this skin-selective mode of action, pimecrolimus has also been shown to impact only minimally on systemic immune responses.[12] This has been demonstrated in a variety of rat models of immunosuppression: the graft *vs* host reaction, antibody formation to sheep red blood cells and an allogenic kidney transplantation model. Thus, systemic administration of pimecrolimus resulted in 8- and 66-fold lower potency in the graft *vs* host reaction than did ciclosporin or tacrolimus respectively. Likewise, tacrolimus was more potent at inhibiting antibody development to sheep red blood cells (48-fold) than pimecrolimus, whilst in the transplantation model pimecrolimus was 3- and 15-fold less potent than ciclosporin and tacrolimus at preventing organ rejection.[12]

> No skin atrophogenic potential was observed with pimecrolimus, in contrast with the corticosteroids which were shown to cause skin atrophy and altered skin texture.

Pimecrolimus
exhibits potent
and skin-selective
anti-inflammatory
activity, with only
a minimal
potential to
suppress systemic
immune
responses.

Thus, these animal studies demonstrate that pimecrolimus exhibits potent and skin-selective anti-inflammatory activity, with only a minimal potential to suppress systemic immune responses.

The skin permeability of pimecrolimus has been compared with tacrolimus *in vitro* in both pig and rat skin.[13] Whilst both compounds permeate into the skin to a similar extent, permeability through the skin was reportedly significantly lower for pimecrolimus than with tacrolimus. Further investigation, using human skin preparations, confirmed the favourable skin penetration/permeation profile of pimecrolimus and showed that the permeation of pimecrolimus through human skin was consistently lower than that of tacrolimus (by a factor of 9–10) and that of the topical corticosteroids, betamethasone valerate, clobetasol propionate and diflucortolon valerate (by a factor of 70–110).[15] This provides further evidence for a lower potential for systemic absorption and thus lower systemic adverse events with pimecrolimus.[13] The differences in permeability are thought to relate to the greater lipophilicity of pimecrolimus compared with tacrolimus.

Pimecrolimus has been shown to inhibit the secondary phase of the immune response (elicitation phase) but not the primary immune response (sensitisation phase) in mice.[16] This contrasts with other immunomodulatory agents used to treat atopic eczema, such as tacrolimus and ciclosporin, which inhibit both phases of the response, and thus, pimecrolimus exerts a more selective immunomodulatory effect. This may be clinically relevant because the elicitation phase represents the clinical manifestation of contact hypersensitivity.[16]

Skin atrophogenic potential

Histological
studies
demonstrated
significant skin
thinning in the
corticosteroid
treatment groups
in contrast to
pimecrolimus and
vehicle treated
subjects.

The lack of skin atrophy associated with pimecrolimus demonstrated in the pig model of allergic contact dermatitis was further confirmed in a human study of 16 healthy volunteers.[17] When pimecrolimus, 1.0%, was applied twice daily to normal skin for 6 days per week in a 4-week randomised, double-blind, vehicle-controlled study, no effects on skin thickness were observed as determined by ultrasound examination. In contrast, after application of the mid-potency topical corticosteroids, betamethasone valerate, 0.1%, and triamcinolone acetonide, 0.1%, skin thickness was significantly reduced by 7.9 and 12.2%, respectively, when compared with baseline. Differences between the treatment groups were significant from treatment day 8 onwards. Moreover, histological studies demonstrated significant skin thinning in the corticosteroid treatment groups in contrast to pimecrolimus and vehicle-treated subjects.

Clinical efficacy

Short-term efficacy in adults

The effectiveness of pimecrolimus cream, 1%, was initially established in patients with moderate atopic eczema in a randomised, double-blind, vehicle-controlled, proof-of-concept study in two comparative areas (right and left arms) of affected skin.[18] A total of 34 adults were randomised to treatment with either a once- or twice-daily application of pimecrolimus, 1.0%, for a total of 3 weeks. To enable a specific evaluation of the effects of pimecrolimus, the vehicle cream was applied at the equivalent affected site on the other arm. However, only small application areas were studied in this preliminary trial (1–2% BSA).

Treatment with twice-daily pimecrolimus cream, 1%, reduced the signs and symptoms of atopic eczema (i.e. erythema, pruritus, exudation, excoriation and lichenification) as determined by the four-point Atopic Dermatitis Severity Index [ADSI]. The mean change in ADSI score from baseline was −71.9% with active treatment compared with −10.3% with vehicle ($p<0.001$). Moreover, improvements in symptoms were observed after only 2 days of treatment (change in ADSI score from baseline: −18.5 vs +1.5%). The median time to partial clearance at the affected site was 8 days. However, once-daily treatment with pimecrolimus was not as effective as twice-daily application (mean reductions in ADSI score from baseline: −37.7 vs −6.2%). When specific symptoms were assessed, in particular pruritus and erythema, the superiority of pimecrolimus was particularly marked. Pimecrolimus was well tolerated in this study, with no rapid rebound of symptoms occurring after discontinuation of the study medication.

As with the earlier pharmacokinetic studies, blood concentrations of pimecrolimus were consistently low in this study, with only two of the 121 samples taken above the limit of quantification (0.1 ng/mL). The authors explain that these samples were the result of treatment contamination of the blood sample during venipuncture.

A double-blind, randomised, parallel-group, multicentre, dose-finding study, evaluated the efficacy of pimecrolimus cream at concentrations of 0.05, 0.2, 0.6 and 1.0%, relative to a matching vehicle control in 260 patients with moderately severe atopic eczema (5–30% BSA).[19] An additional internal control was also employed, in which a subgroup of patients received the mid-potency topical corticosteroid, betamethasone valerate, 0.1%. All treatments were administered twice daily for up to 3 weeks. The primary endpoint of the study was change from baseline in an adapted Eczema Area Severity Index (EASI), which assessed the key symptoms of atopic eczema on a four-point scale (ranging from zero, representing no clinical sign, to three for severe expression). The effects of the different treatment regimens on pruritus were also evaluated. Finally, patients were asked to record their perception of symptom improvement at the end of the study.

The median EASI score decreased significantly over the course of the study in a dose-dependent fashion in the pimecrolimus, 0.2, 0.6 and 1.0% treatment groups (p-values vs placebo: 0.041, 0.001 and 0.008). The greatest reductions in the EASI score were seen in patients who received betamethasone valerate, followed by those who received pimecrolimus, 1.0 and 0.6%. However, as predicted, no significant effect on the EASI score was observed with the lowest dose of pimecrolimus (0.05%). Pruritus was also significantly improved in the pimecrolimus, 0.2, 0.6 and 1.0%, treatment groups, with greater proportions of patients rating pruritus as mild or absent compared with vehicle

> Treatment with twice-daily pimecrolimus cream, 1%, reduced the signs and symptoms of atopic eczema as determined by the Atopic Dermatitis Severity Index.

> The median EASI score decreased significantly over the course of the study in a dose-dependent fashion in the pimecrolimus, 0.2, 0.6 and 1.0%, treatment groups.

(Table 1). Again, corticosteroid treatment was more effective in reducing pruritus relative to any pimecrolimus dose. When patients rated their own response to treatment, greater proportions of patients in the pimecrolimus, 1.0, 0.6 and 0.2% treatment groups reported their symptoms to be moderately clear or better compared with vehicle (53.3, 54.8 and 32.6%, respectively, *vs* 16.3% with vehicle). As with the other efficacy endpoints, patients receiving betamethasone valerate reported the highest rate of symptomatic improvement (88.1%).

Pimecrolimus was well tolerated in this study, with no systemic adverse events reported that were attributable to active treatment. The principal local adverse events were application site reactions (i.e. burning, feeling of warmth, stinging, smarting, pain and soreness), which were generally transient and resolved within 3 days of treatment at the 1.0% dose. Overall, the incidence of adverse events were similar in all the pimecrolimus treatment groups.

Thus, in conclusion, pimecrolimus was well tolerated and effective in improving the symptoms of atopic eczema, including pruritus, in adult patients. The 1.0% dose exerted the greatest therapeutic effect amongst the pimecrolimus treatment groups and had the best tolerability profile amongst the different range of doses tested, and thus, this dose was selected for further testing in phase 3 clinical studies.

Short-term efficacy in children

Two multicentre, randomised, double-blind, vehicle-controlled studies have examined the short-term efficacy of pimecrolimus cream, 1%, in paediatric patients (n=403; aged 2–18 years; mean age: 6.7 years) with mostly moderate atopic eczema.[20] As both studies were of similar design and had similar entry requirements, the data generated from them were pooled.

Table 1. Proportion of patients with absent or mild pruritus (defined as a score of zero or one respectively, in a dose-ranging study of pimecrolimus cream, with an internal control of betamethasone valerate.[19]

Treatment group	Percentage of patients with absent or mild pruritus		
	Baseline	Day 8	Day 22
Vehicle	4.7	14.0	18.6
Pimecrolimus, 0.05%	4.8	4.8	23.8
Pimecrolimus, 0.2%	8.7	23.9	37.0
Pimecrolimus, 0.6%	11.9	23.8	52.4
Pimecrolimus, 1.0%	6.7	40.0	46.7
Betamethasone valerate	11.9	78.6	81.0

Both studies employed the Investigators Global Assessment (IGA) at each study visit to evaluate response to study treatment. The IGA assesses disease severity according to morphology without reference to baseline status, and ranks severity on a six-point scale, where zero represents clear and five is very severe. On entry, patients were required to have an IGA score of between two and three. The percentage of patients who achieved an IGA score of zero or one (clear or almost clear) was the primary endpoint of both studies. Additional assessments included change from baseline in EASI score, severity of pruritus and patient/caregiver assessment of overall disease control.

Patients were randomised 2:1 to receive pimecrolimus, 1%, or vehicle, applied twice daily for 6 weeks. In the pooled analysis, after 6 weeks of treatment, 34.8% of patients receiving pimecrolimus, 1.0%, had IGA scores of zero or one (representing clear or almost clear of disease signs) compared with 18.4% who received vehicle ($p \leq 0.05$; Figure 3). Pimecrolimus had a rapid onset of action, exemplified by an early improvement in symptoms, with a clear and significant difference between treatment groups observed at the first evaluation visit on day 8 (12.0 vs 2.2%, respectively; $p \leq 0.05$ [Figure 3]). In terms of treatment response assessed by the EASI, significant improvements were also observed with pimecrolimus, 1%, relative to the vehicle, and these improvements paralleled the improvements seen in the IGA. The maximum response on this measure of efficacy was observed by day 29 (–47 vs +1%, respectively; $p \leq 0.001$) and this effect was maintained until the end of the study (Figure 4). When the EASI score for the face and

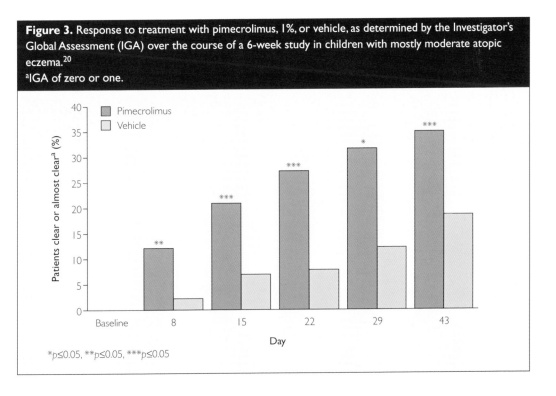

Figure 3. Response to treatment with pimecrolimus, 1%, or vehicle, as determined by the Investigator's Global Assessment (IGA) over the course of a 6-week study in children with mostly moderate atopic eczema.[20]
[a]IGA of zero or one.

*$p \leq 0.05$, **$p \leq 0.05$, ***$p \leq 0.05$

Figure 4. Response to treatment with pimecrolimus, 1%, or vehicle, as determined by the Eczema Area Severity Index (EASI) over the course of a 6-week study in children with mostly moderate atopic eczema.[20]

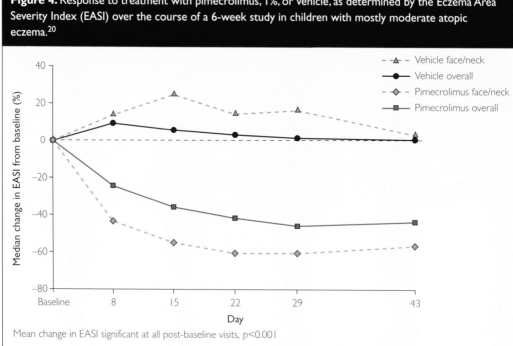

Mean change in EASI significant at all post-baseline visits, $p < 0.001$

neck region was monitored, more profound reductions were observed with pimecrolimus, 1% (Figure 4). Pruritus was also significantly improved in patients who received pimecrolimus. Significantly more patients receiving active treatment reported mild or no pruritus than those who received vehicle. Again, this effect was observed early in the study and was maintained throughout its duration. In terms of patient/carer's perception of efficacy, significantly more patients receiving pimecrolimus than vehicle reported complete or good disease control.

Another secondary assessment of these studies was the impact of treatment upon the quality of life of patients.[21] These analyses included patients aged 8 years of age or younger from the entire patient cohort. Evaluations were made using the Parent's Index of Quality of Life in Atopic Dermatitis (PIQoL-AD) tool in which the parent or caregiver of the patient assesses the improvements in the child's quality of life. Both the pimecrolimus and control groups reported improved quality of life from baseline, although the improvements with pimecrolimus were significantly greater after 6 weeks' treatment. At the end of the 6-week blinded period of the studies, all patients in the control group were switched to open-label pimecrolimus treatment. This led to equivalent PIQoL-AD scores in both treatment groups at the end of 6 months' treatment.

Thus, in conclusion, treatment with pimecrolimus cream, 1%, significantly improved the symptoms of atopic eczema in children aged 2–18 years, in comparison with the vehicle control, and had a rapid onset of action, with significant improvements in all efficacy parameters

> Treatment with pimecrolimus significantly improved the symptoms of atopic eczema in children aged 2–18 years.

observed by the first study visit, 8 days after the start of the study. These improvements provide significant and beneficial effects on patients' quality of life. There has been some criticism as to why these pooled studies did not report the individual data from each study population, in addition to combining them in one pooled analysis, and also of other elements of the study design and its reporting.[22] However, many of these criticisms have been resolved in a recent response by the authors of this study.[23]

Impact of baseline factors on treatment outcomes

A pooled analysis of data derived from the short-term paediatric trials of pimecrolimus, 1%, included 589 children (186 of whom were aged under 23 months at randomisation and as such, are outside the UK licensed indication for pimecrolimus).[24] Study participants were first stratified, according to their ethnic origin, into Caucasian and non-Caucasian groups (55 and 45% of the total study population, respectively). The rate of treatment success, judged in terms of changes in IGA and EASI scores, was significantly higher in children receiving pimecrolimus than in those receiving vehicle, regardless of ethnic origin. The proportions of Caucasian patients with an IGA score of zero or one (clear or almost clear) after 43 days of treatment were 45 and 23.6% for pimecrolimus and vehicle, respectively (p=0.02), whilst the corresponding proportions of non-Caucasian patients were 36.3 and 15.7%, respectively (p<0.001). Similarly, the differences between pimecrolimus and vehicle, as evaluated using the EASI scale, were –4.35 and –5.37 for Caucasian and non-Caucasian patients, respectively (p<0.001 *vs* vehicle for both comparisons). The tolerability of pimecrolimus was also unaffected by ethnic origin, such that the overall incidence of application site burning was low and comparable between ethnic groups (9.0 and 7.1% for Caucasian and non-Caucasian groups, respectively; p=0.45).

Analysis of the pooled data on the basis of disease severity at baseline also revealed no differences in treatment outcome following pimecrolimus treatment. Thus, patients with mild (IGA of two) or moderate (IGA of three) disease severity at baseline demonstrated similar treatment effects (absolute differences of 19.2 and 23.3%, respectively; p<0.01 *vs* vehicle). However, there were too few patients with severe or very severe disease to permit useful comparisons.

Overall, these data indicate that neither ethnic origin nor baseline disease severity affected patients' response to pimecrolimus in short-term efficacy studies.

> Neither ethnic origin nor baseline disease severity affected patients' response to pimecrolimus in short-term efficacy studies.

Long-term prevention of disease flare progression in adults

A long-term randomised, double-blind, parallel-group, multicentre study, assessed whether treatment with pimecrolimus, 1%, applied at the first sign or symptom of atopic eczema would prevent progression to disease flares[a] and thus reduce the need for topical corticosteroids, the standard treatment regimen in such instances.[25] A total of 192 adults with moderate-to-severe atopic eczema (mean BSA: 17%; IGA score: three or four) were randomised to treatment with either pimecrolimus, 1%, or vehicle, applied as required for 24 weeks. If disease flares occurred, a moderate-potency corticosteroid, prednicarbate, 0.25%, was permitted as rescue therapy in both treatment groups. The primary endpoint of the study was the proportion of days on which prednicarbate was required to control disease flares. Other outcome measures included the number of disease flares, time to first flare, IGA and EASI scores, pruritus severity, and patients' self-assessment.

Treatment with pimecrolimus, 1%, led to a significant reduction in the percentage of days on which prednicarbate treatment was applied, compared with vehicle (14.2 *vs* 37.2% of study days, respectively; $p<0.001$). Almost half (49%) of the patients who received pimecrolimus, 1%, did not require any corticosteroid treatment over the duration of the study, compared with 22% in the control group. Significantly fewer disease flares occurred after treatment with pimecrolimus (mean of 1.1 *vs* 2.4 flares in the pimecrolimus and vehicle groups, respectively; $p<0.0001$) whilst the time to first disease flare was also longer with the active treatment (median time to first flare: 144 *vs* 26 days).

With regard to the other efficacy parameters, pimecrolimus provided significant improvements in disease symptoms as assessed by the IGA, reduced the severity of pruritus, reduced the mean EASI score and reduced the extent of the area of body surface affected more favourably than those who received the vehicle control (Table 2). Moreover, the improvement in symptoms of atopic eczema that occurred with active treatment provided significant improvements in the quality of life of patients during the course of the study as demonstrated by reductions in the QoL Index – Atopic Dermatitis (QoLIAD) scale (−25.6 *vs* −7.4%; $p=0.002$) and in the Dermatology Life Quality Index (DLQI) score (−22.0 *vs* −6.7%; $p=0.01$) (Table 2).

Pimecrolimus was well tolerated in this study, with a similar incidence of adverse events in the active and control treatment groups (24.0 *vs* 20.8%). The principal drug-related adverse event was application site burning which occurred more frequently in the pimecrolimus group (10 cases *vs* 3 cases in the vehicle group). However, these events were transient and resolved within 7 days.

In conclusion, this study has demonstrated that pimecrolimus, 1%, has the potential to reduce the need for topical corticosteroids to treat disease flares when given at the first signs or symptoms of atopic eczema in adult patients. This novel treatment strategy may allow corticosteroid therapy to be reserved for rescue therapy only, thereby reducing their long-term use and minimising steroid-associated side-effects.

Pimecrolimus has the potential to reduce the need for topical corticosteroids to treat disease flares when given at the first signs or symptoms of atopic eczema in adult patients.

---

[a]Defined as disease status requiring topical corticosteroid therapy for at least 3 days.

Table 2. Studies of pimecrolimus, 1%, compared with vehicle, in the long-term prevention of disease flares in patients with moderate-to-severe atopic eczema.[25,26]

Study	Main outcomes
Meurer et al., 2002[25] Randomised, double-blind, multicentre, parallel-group, vehicle-controlled, 24-week study n=192 adults with moderate-to severe atopic eczema (IGA score: three or four).	• Corticosteroid rescue was significantly less frequent with pimecrolimus compared with vehicle (14.2 vs 37.2% of study days; $p<0.001$) • There was no requirement for corticosteroid rescue in almost half of the pimecrolimus-treated patients (49%), compared with 21.9% in the control group. • The incidence of disease flares was lower with pimecrolimus (mean incidence: 1.1 vs 2.4; $p<0.001$). In total, 44.8% of patients experienced no flare with pimecrolimus, compared with 18.8% receiving vehicle. • The median time to first flare was significantly longer with pimecrolimus than with vehicle (144 vs 26 days; $p<0.001$). • The symptoms of atopic eczema were significantly improved with pimecrolimus compared with vehicle as assessed by the IGA, EASI and patient self-assessment (IGA score of ≤two: 68.6 vs 36.5%; EASI: −48.3 vs −15.9%; $p<0.001$; patient assessment: 64.6 vs 35.4%). • The pruritus score was reduced with pimecrolimus within the first 2 days of treatment and was significantly different from the vehicle-controlled group from day 3 onwards ($p<0.001$). • The improvement in quality of life was significantly greater in the pimecrolimus group than those in the control group as assessed by the QoLIAD ($p=0.002$) and DLQI ($p=0.01$) scores. • Pimecrolimus was well-tolerated with a similar incidence of adverse events in the active and control treatment groups (24.0 vs 20.8%). Application site burning occurred more frequently with active treatment (10 vs 3 cases).
Wahn et al., 2002[26] Randomised, double-blind, vehicle-controlled, 1-year study n=713 children (aged 2–17 years) with moderate atopic eczema	• There were significantly fewer disease flares amongst patients treated with pimecrolimus compared with vehicle, regardless of disease severity. Thus, severely affected patients also benefited from treatment. • Approximately twice as many patients who received pimecrolimus reported no disease flares compared with those in the vehicle group (6 months' treatment: 61.0 vs 34.2%; 12 months' treatment: 50.8 vs 28.3%). • Pimecrolimus treatment was associated with a significantly longer flare-free period. • Fewer patients who received pimecrolimus required topical corticosteroid rescue therapy compared with the vehicle control group (6 months' treatment: 35.0 vs 62.9%; 12 months' treatment: 42.6 vs 68.4%) whilst fewer days were spent on rescue therapy with pimecrolimus treatment (1–14 days: 17.1 vs 27.5%; >14 days 25.5 vs 41.0%).

QoLIAD, Quality of Life Index – Atopic Dermatitis; DLQI, Dermatology Life Quality Index.

Table 2. Continued	
Study	Main outcomes
Wahn *et al.*, 2002[26] *(continued)*	• Median EASI scores and IGA scores were lower in the pimecrolimus group over the course of the study than in the control group. • The incidence of adverse events in both treatment groups were similar and not significantly different (24.7% with pimecrolimus *vs* 18.7% with control). The most common adverse event was a sensation of burning (10.5 *vs* 9.3%, pimecrolimus *vs* control). Skin infections were similar in both groups. However, the incidence of grouped viral skin infections was slightly higher in the pimecrolimus group compared with control (12.4 *vs* 6.3%).

QoLIAD, Quality of Life Index – Atopic Dermatitis; DLQI, Dermatology Life Quality Index.

Long-term prevention of disease flare progression in children

A study of broadly similar design has investigated long-term disease control with pimecrolimus, 1%, compared with standard treatment (emollients and topical corticosteroids) in children with mostly moderate atopic eczema.[26] This study differed from the adult trial discussed previously in that it had a 12-month treatment duration and enrolled patients with mild-to-moderate atopic eczema. The principal objective was to determine whether pimecrolimus, 1%, applied at the first sign or symptom of atopic eczema, could prevent the progression to disease flares, and thus influence long-term clinical outcome. This was a 1-year, randomised, double-blind, vehicle-controlled study of 713 paediatric patients with atopic eczema (aged 2–17 years; mean age 8 years). Patients were randomised to pimecrolimus or vehicle as necessary to treat early signs or symptoms of atopic eczema. If flares occurred, a moderately potent topical corticosteroid was applied. Emollients were also used in both groups to control dry skin. The primary endpoint of the study was ranked flares at 6 months' follow-up.

> Approximately twice as many patients in the pimecrolimus group than in the control group completed 6 or 12 months' treatment without any disease flares.

This study reported fewer disease flares after pimecrolimus treatment compared with those in the control group (incidence data not reported). Approximately twice as many patients in the pimecrolimus group than in the control group completed 6 or 12 months' treatment without any disease flares (Figure 5). The greater control of disease flares with pimecrolimus was maintained irrespective of baseline atopic eczema severity. The time to first disease flare was significantly longer in the pimecrolimus group. Consequently, fewer patients required corticosteroid rescue than those receiving vehicle (6 months: 35.0 *vs* 62.9%; 12 months: 42.6 *vs* 68.4%) whilst more patients receiving pimecrolimus did not require any corticosteroid treatment than those who received topical corticosteroids over the 12 months of the study (57.4 *vs* 31.6%). Other measures of efficacy also demonstrated the

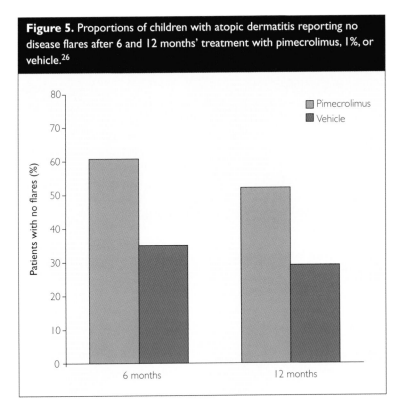

Figure 5. Proportions of children with atopic dermatitis reporting no disease flares after 6 and 12 months' treatment with pimecrolimus, 1%, or vehicle.[26]

superior control of atopic eczema with the pimecrolimus treatment regimen. Thus, the median EASI scores were consistently lower in the pimecrolimus group, whilst the responses on the IGA also supported superior control with pimecrolimus. All the efficacy data from this study are summarised in Table 2.

Again pimecrolimus was well tolerated, with a similar incidence of adverse events in both treatment groups. Application site reactions were the most common adverse events, although there were no differences between treatment groups in this regard. There were also no significant differences between treatment groups with respect to local skin infections, although there was a slightly higher incidence associated with pimecrolimus when the incidence of viral skin infections were grouped together (12.4 *vs* 6.3%).

In conclusion, pimecrolimus was effective in preventing progression of disease flares when applied at the first sign or symptom of atopic eczema in children with moderate atopic eczema, and thus treatment with pimecrolimus had a steroid-sparing effect in this patient population. The effects of pimecrolimus were apparent at 6 months, and this effect was maintained over 12 months.

A number of other clinical studies have reported which have demonstrated short-term[27] and long-term[28] efficacy of pimecrolimus, 1%, in infants and in other inflammatory skin disorders including contact dermatitis,[29] hand dermatitis[30] and psoriasis.[31,32] However, as pimecrolimus is not indicated for these conditions or recommended for

> Pimecrolimus was effective in preventing progression of disease flares when applied at the first sign or symptom of atopic eczema in children with moderate atopic eczema.

use in children under 2 years, it is beyond the scope of this review to discuss these data here.

Comparative studies

The first randomised clinical trial that directly compared the relative efficacy and safety of pimecrolimus and tacrolimus, was conducted in a group of 141 paediatric patients with moderately severe atopic eczema, aged 2–17 years.[33] Children were randomly allocated to 6 weeks' treatment with either pimecrolimus cream (1%) or tacrolimus ointment (0.03%), with the primary evaluation being the relative local tolerability of each agent. After 4 days of administration, the rate of erythema or irritation was significantly lower amongst pimecrolimus- than tacrolimus-treated patients (8 *vs* 19%, respectively; *p*=0.039). Furthermore, the proportion of tacrolimus-treated patients experiencing erythema or irritation persisting for longer than 30 minutes was significantly higher than the corresponding proportion of pimecrolimus patients (85 *vs* 0%, respectively; *p*<0.001). In terms of efficacy, the two treatments were judged to be equally effective. The proportions of patients in each treatment group achieving IGA scores of clear/almost clear (i.e. scores of zero or one) after 43 days were statistically similar (30 *vs* 42% for pimecrolimus and tacrolimus, respectively; *p*=0.119).

The patient- or caregiver-assessed acceptability scores for each treatment are presented in Figure 6. As can be seen from the figure, pimecrolimus was consistently rated as very good or excellent by a higher proportion of patients than was tacrolimus, particularly in terms of its suitability for use on facial skin and its ease of application (*p*=0.009 and *p*=0.02, respectively).

> Pimecrolimus was consistently rated as very good or excellent by a higher proportion of patients than was tacrolimus, particularly in terms of its suitability for use on facial skin and its ease of application.

Meta-analyses

Currently, two meta-analyses of published randomised controlled trials have indirectly compared the effectiveness of pimecrolimus and tacrolimus in the treatment of atopic dermatitis.[34,35] Both comparisons included only those randomised controlled trials that compared licensed therapeutic doses of either of the two agents with vehicle or another active treatment.

In the first analysis, which included 25 trials and incorporated 4186 and 6897 patients treated with pimecrolimus and tacrolimus, respectively, both agents were reported to be significantly more effective than vehicle.[34] Tacrolimus (0.1%) was shown to be as effective as potent topical corticosteroids (e.g. hydrocortisone butyrate, 0.1%, betamethasone valerate, 0.1%) and also more effective than mild topical corticosteroids (e.g. hydrocortisone acetate, 1%) in treating atopic eczema. In contrast, pimecrolimus (1%) was less effective than betamethasone valerate (1%) after 3 weeks and has not been compared with mild topical corticosteroids. The single study that directly compared pimecrolimus with tacrolimus was discussed previously.

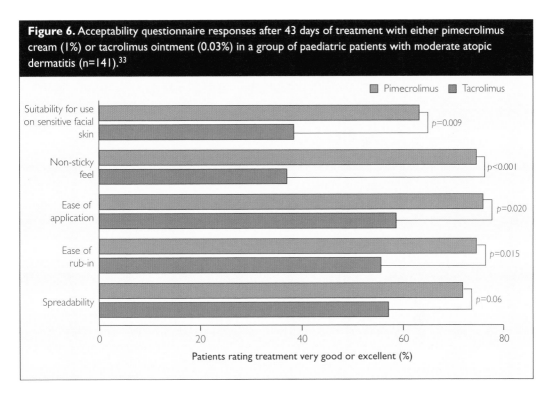

Figure 6. Acceptability questionnaire responses after 43 days of treatment with either pimecrolimus cream (1%) or tacrolimus ointment (0.03%) in a group of paediatric patients with moderate atopic dermatitis (n=141).[33]

The second analysis included a smaller number of trials (n=16) and thus a more condensed patient population (1225 pimecrolimus-, 2107 tacrolimus- and 1969 vehicle-treated patients).[35] The tacrolimus group contained a greater proportion of patients with severe atopic dermatitis than the pimecrolimus group, which may have impacted on overall outcomes (48.7 *vs* 13.9%, respectively; *p*-value not reported). Furthermore, the pimecrolimus studies were generally of longer duration than those of tacrolimus (up to 12 months compared with up to 3 months). Overall, pimecrolimus reduced EASI scores by 61.5% after 1 month of treatment, compared with a reduction of 65.6% following tacrolimus at the same time point (*p*-value not reported). At 6 and 12 months, the score reductions associated with pimecrolimus treatment were 61.5 and 60.3%, respectively. Since the tacrolimus studies did not extend beyond 3 months (at which point the score reduction was 73%) further comparisons cannot be made. In general, the success rates associated with the two drugs were statistically similar, although tacrolimus was used in patients with more severe disease at baseline. These analyses underline the need for further head-to-head comparisons of pimecrolimus and tacrolimus, before any definitive conclusions regarding comparative efficacy can be made.

Safety and tolerability

Topical pimecrolimus is generally well tolerated when used in both adults and children. As discussed, the principal adverse event associated

You are strongly urged to consult your doctor before taking, stopping or changing any of the products reviewed or referred to in *BESTMEDICINE* or any other medication that has been prescribed or recommended by your doctor.

with its use was a mild-to-moderate local skin irritation (described as a moderate burning, warmth or stinging sensation) at the application site, which generally resolved within 3 days of treatment. It occurs in approximately 15 and 7% of treated adults and children, respectively.[36] However, meta-analyses suggest that there are no differences in the incidence of application site irritation between pimecrolimus and the vehicle, suggesting that this side-effect may not necessarily derive from the active agent.[36] Interestingly, the incidence of application site irritation appears to be lower with pimecrolimus than with topical tacrolimus.[37] Given the low systemic exposure to pimecrolimus after topical administration, no clinically relevant systemic adverse events have been recorded in patients with atopic eczema who were treated with pimecrolimus. Most notably, and as discussed previously, no skin atrophy has been observed with pimecrolimus, in contrast with corticosteroids.[17]

> Most notably no skin atrophy has been observed with pimecrolimus, in contrast with corticosteroids.

The principal concerns relating to pimecrolimus treatment are focused on impairment of local skin immunosurveillance, leading to possible increases in local infections and a potential for an increased risk of skin cancer. Further, long-term safety data are required to exclude or confirm this link. However, the incidence of fungal and viral infections was not significantly increased with pimecrolimus treatment in the clinical trial programme, whilst bacterial infection was lower with pimecrolimus than the vehicle control, probably due to the parallel improvement in eczematous lesions with active treatment.[31] In cases where pre-existing cutaneous viral infections exist, pimecrolimus should not be applied until the localised infection clears.[11]

Drug–drug interactions with pimecrolimus would be expected to be minimal, given the low systemic availability of pimecrolimus. However, as pimecrolimus is metabolised by CYP 3A4, coadministration with known inhibitors of this isoenzyme (e.g. erythromycin, itraconazole, ketoconazole, fluconazole, calcium-channel blockers and cimetidine) should be performed with caution.

Long-term safety data

A long-term, double-blind study in 658 adults with moderate-to-severe atopic eczema, compared the safety and tolerability profile of pimecrolimus cream, 1%, with that of the topical corticosteroids, triamcinolone acetonide, 1%, and hydrocortisone acetate, 1%.[38] Patients applied their respective treatments twice daily to all affected areas and continued treatment over a 1-year period until inflammation had cleared completely. The majority of patients continued drug treatment for 1 year, such that the median percentages of days of exposure to study medication were 99.5 and 95.6% for pimecrolimus and topical corticosteroids, respectively (*p*-value not reported). In patients with at least 30% of their body surface area affected by atopic eczema, the incidence of all skin infections (including bacterial, fungal and herpes infections) was significantly lower following treatment with pimecrolimus than topical corticosteroids (treatment difference –25.3 to

−3.4%; *p*-values not reported). The most common systemic adverse events associated with active treatment were nasopharyngitis (7.6 *vs* 13.9% for pimecrolimus and topical corticosteroids, respectively; *p*-value not reported) and influenza (9.8 *vs* 11.5%, respectively; *p*-value not reported). The most frequently reported application site reaction was burning, which affected 25.9% of pimecrolimus- and 10.9% of corticosteroid-treated patients, respectively (*p*-value not reported). The majority of adverse events were transient and of mild-to-moderate intensity and no clinically significant systemic adverse events were reported for either treatment.

Key points

● Pimecrolimus is a cell-specific inhibitor of cytokine expression and release from activated T cells – a major component in the aetiology of atopic eczema.

● Pimecrolimus is not absorbed systemically, with blood levels remaining consistently low in a variety of patient populations. This lack of systemic absorption reduces the likelihood of significant drug–drug interactions and adverse systemic immune suppression.

● Preclinical studies have demonstrated that pimecrolimus binds with high affinity to the cytosolic macrophillin-12 molecule, in a similar fashion to tacrolimus and ciclosporin. This prevents the transcription of various cytokines from activated T cells. In addition, pimecrolimus prevents the release of preformed pro-inflammatory mediators from mast cells.

● Animal models of inflammatory skin disorders have demonstrated the potent and selective anti-inflammatory and immunomodulating effects of pimecrolimus. Moreover, unlike topical corticosteroids, pimecrolimus has no skin atrophogenic potential, as demonstrated in both animal studies and in human volunteers.

● The potent anti-inflammatory effects appear to be localised to skin tissue, with minimal effects on systemic immune response – an important pharmacological profile for a topical anti-inflammatory agent.

● A large clinical trial programme has demonstrated that pimecrolimus is effective in both the short-term treatment of atopic eczema and the prevention of progression to disease flares in both adults and children, and thus can reduce the need for topical corticosteroid rescue therapy when used at the first sign or symptom of the condition.

● Pimecrolimus is generally well tolerated in both adults and children. The principal adverse event that occurs is a local application site irritation, which is mild-to-moderate in intensity but which usually resolves within 3 days of treatment.

References

A list of the published evidence which has been reviewed in compiling the preceding section of *BESTMEDICINE*.

1 Charman C, Morris A, Williams H. Topical steroid phobia in dermatology outpatients with atopic eczema. *Br J Dermatol* 1999; **141(Suppl 55)**: 105.

2 Grassberger M, Baumruker T, Enz A *et al*. A novel anti-inflammatory drug, SDZ ASM 981, for the treatment of skin diseases: *in vitro* pharmacology. *Br J Dermatol* 1999; **141**: 264–73.

3 Wellington K, Jarvis B. Spotlight on topical pimecrolimus in atopic dermatitis. *Am J Clin Dermatol* 2002; **3**: 435–8.

4 Zuberbier T, Chong SU, Grunow K *et al*. The ascomycin macrolactam pimecrolimus (Elidel, SDZ ASM 981) is a potent inhibitor of mediator release from human dermal mast cells and peripheral blood basophils. *J Allergy Clin Immunol* 2001; **108**: 275–80.

5 Hultsch T, Muller KD, Meingassner JG *et al*. Ascomycin macrolactam derivative SDZ ASM 981 inhibits the release of granule-associated mediators and of newly synthesized cytokines in RBL 2H3 mast cells in an immunophilin-dependent manner. *Arch Dermatol Res* 1998; **290**: 501–7.

6 Kalthoff FS, Chung J, Stuetz A. Pimecrolimus inhibits up-regulation of OX40 and synthesis of inflammatory cytokines upon secondary T-cell activation by allogeneic dendritic cells. *Clin Exp Immunol* 2002; **130**: 85–92.

7 Meingassner JG, Kowalsky E, Schwendinger H, Elbe-Burger A, Stutz A. Pimecrolimus does not affect Langerhans cells in murine epidermis. *Br J Dermatol* 2003; **149**: 853–7.

8 Van Leent EJ, Ebelin ME, Burtin P *et al*. Low systemic exposure after repeated topical application of Pimecrolimus (Elidel, SDZ ASM 981) in patients with atopic dermatitis. *Dermatology* 2002; **204**: 63–8.

9 Harper J, Green A, Scott G *et al*. First experience of topical SDZ ASM 981 in children with atopic dermatitis. *Br J Dermatol* 2001; **144**: 781–7.

10 Allen BR, Lakhanpaul M, Morris A *et al*. Systemic exposure, tolerability, and efficacy of pimecrolimus cream 1% in atopic dermatitis patients. *Arch Dis Child* 2003; **88**: 969–73.

11 Novartis Pharmaceuticals UK Ltd. Elidel® (pimecrolimus) cream 1%. *Summary of product characteristics*. Camberley, Surrey, 2003.

12 Meingassner JG, Grassberger M, Fahrngruber H *et al*. A novel anti-inflammatory drug, SDZ ASM 981, for the topical and oral treatment of skin diseases: *in vivo* pharmacology. *Br J Dermatol* 1997; **137**: 568–76.

13 Stuetz A, Grassberger M, Meingassner JG. Pimecrolimus (Elidel, SDZ ASM 981) – preclinical pharmacologic profile and skin selectivity. *Semin Cutan Med Surg* 2001; **20**: 233–41.

14 Neckermann G, Bavandi A, Meingassner JG. Atopic dermatitis-like symptoms in hypomagnesaemic hairless rats are prevented and inhibited by systemic or topical SDZ ASM 981. *Br J Dermatol* 2000; **142**: 669–79.

15 Billich A, Aschauer H, Aszodi A, Stuetz A. Percutaneous absorption of drugs used in atopic eczema: pimecrolimus permeates less through skin than corticosteroids and tacrolimus. *Int J Pharm* 2004; **269**: 29–35.

16 Meingassner JG, Fahrngruber H, Bavandi A. Pimecrolimus inhibits the elicitation phase but does not suppress the sensitization phase in murine contact hypersensitivity, in contrast to tacrolimus and cyclosporine A. *J Invest Dermatol* 2003; **121**: 77–80.

17 Queille-Roussel C, Paul C, Duteil L *et al*. The new topical ascomycin derivative SDZ ASM 981 does not induce skin atrophy when applied to normal skin for 4 weeks: a randomized, double-blind controlled study. *Br J Dermatol* 2001; **144**: 507–13.

18 Van Leent EJ, Graber M, Thurston M *et al*. Effectiveness of the ascomycin macrolactam SDZ ASM 981 in the topical treatment of atopic dermatitis. *Arch Dermatol* 1998; **134**: 805–9.

19 Luger T, Van Leent EJ, Graeber M *et al*. SDZ ASM 981: an emerging safe and effective treatment for atopic dermatitis. *Br J Dermatol* 2001; **144**: 788–94.

20 Eichenfield LF, Lucky AW, Boguniewicz M *et al*. Safety and efficacy of pimecrolimus (ASM 981) cream 1% in the treatment of mild and moderate atopic dermatitis in children and adolescents. *J Am Acad Dermatol* 2002; **46**: 495–504.

21 Whalley D, Huels J, McKenna SP, Van Assche D. The benefit of pimecrolimus (Elidel, SDZ ASM 981) on parents' quality of life in the treatment of pediatric atopic dermatitis. *Pediatrics* 2002; **110**: 1133–6.

22 Williams H. Another vehicle-controlled study of 1% pimecrolimus in atopic dermatitis: how does it help clinicians and patients, and is it ethically sound? *Arch Dermatol* 2002; **138**: 1602–3.

23 Eichenfield LF, Lucky AW, Boguniewicz M *et al*. 1% pimecrolimus cream for atopic dermatitis. *Arch Dermatol* 2003; **139**: 1369–70; author reply 70–1.

24 Eichenfield L, Lucky A, Langley R *et al*. Use of pimecrolimus cream 1% (Elidel) in the treatment of atopic dermatitis in infants and children: the effects of ethnic origin and baseline disease severity on treatment outcome. *Int J Dermatol* 2005; **44**: 70–5.

25 Meurer M, Folster-Holst R, Wozel G *et al*. Pimecrolimus cream in the long-term management of atopic dermatitis in adults: a six-month study. *Dermatology* 2002; **205**: 271–7.

26 Wahn U, Bos JD, Goodfield M *et al*. Efficacy and safety of pimecrolimus cream in the long-term management of atopic dermatitis in children. *Pediatrics* 2002; **110**: e2.

27 Ho VC, Gupta A, Kaufmann R *et al*. Safety and efficacy of nonsteroid pimecrolimus cream 1% in the treatment of atopic dermatitis in infants. *J Pediatr* 2003; **142**: 155–62.

28 Kapp A, Papp K, Bingham A *et al.* Long-term management of atopic dermatitis in infants with topical pimecrolimus, a nonsteroid anti-inflammatory drug. *J Allergy Clin Immunol* 2002; **110**: 277–84.

29 Queille-Roussel C, Graeber M, Thurston M *et al.* SDZ ASM 981 is the first non-steroid that suppresses established nickel contact dermatitis elicited by allergen challenge. *Contact Dermatitis* 2000; **42**: 349–50.

30 Thaci D, Steinmeyer K, Ebelin ME, Scott G, Kaufmann R. Occlusive treatment of chronic hand dermatitis with pimecrolimus cream 1% results in low systemic exposure, is well tolerated, safe, and effective. An open study. *Dermatology* 2003; **207**: 37–42.

31 Mrowietz U, Graeber M, Brautigam M *et al.* The novel ascomycin derivative SDZ ASM 981 is effective for psoriasis when used topically under occlusion. *Br J Dermatol* 1998; **139**: 992–6.

32 Mrowietz U, Wustlich S, Hoexter G *et al.* An experimental ointment formulation of pimecrolimus is effective in psoriasis without occlusion. *Acta Derm Venereol* 2003; **83**: 351–3.

33 Kempers S, Boguniewicz M, Carter E *et al.* A randomized investigator-blinded study comparing pimecrolimus cream 1% with tacrolimus ointment 0.03% in the treatment of pediatric patients with moderate atopic dermatitis. *J Am Acad Dermatol* 2004; **51**: 515–25.

34 Ashcroft D, Dimmock P, Garside R, Stein K, Williams H. Efficacy and tolerability of topical pimecrolimus and tacrolimus in the treatment of atopic dermatitis: meta-analysis of randomised controlled trials. *BMJ* 2005; **330**: 516.

35 Iskedjian M, Piwko C, Shear N, Langley R, Einarson T. Topical calcineurin inhibitors in the treatment of atopic dermatitis: a meta-analysis of current evidence. *Am J Clin Dermatol* 2004; **5**: 267–79.

36 Graham-Brown RA, Grassberger M. Pimecrolimus: a review of pre-clinical and clinical data. *Int J Clin Pract* 2003; **57**: 319–27.

37 Nghiem P, Pearson G, Langley RG. Tacrolimus and pimecrolimus: from clever prokaryotes to inhibiting calcineurin and treating atopic dermatitis. *J Am Acad Dermatol* 2002; **46**: 228–41.

38 Luger T, Lahfa M, Folster-Holst R *et al.* Long-term safety and tolerability of pimecrolimus cream 1% and topical corticosteroids in adults with moderate to severe atopic dermatitis. *J Dermatolog Treat* 2004; **15**: 169–78.

Acknowledgements

Figures 3 and 4 are adapted from Eichenfield *et al.*, 2002.[20]

Figure 5 is adapted from Wahn *et al.*, 2002.[26]

Figure 6 is adapted from Kempers *et al.*, 2004.[33]

4. Drug review – Tacrolimus (Protopic®)

Dr Anna Palmer
CSF Medical Communications Ltd

Summary

Tacrolimus was developed in the 1990s as a topical immunomodulatory therapy for atopic eczema. Tacrolimus was originally developed as a systemic immunosuppressant to prevent rejection of organ transplants, and continues to be used in this way. As a topical ointment formulation, tacrolimus exhibits minimal systemic absorption and no systemic accumulation. This property ensures an excellent tolerability profile, with side-effects limited to mild local irritation. The most common adverse events are sensations of skin burning and itching, and these symptoms tend to disappear as the skin heals, generally within a matter of days. Clinical trials conducted over the short- and long-term in both adults and in children aged over 2 years have shown that tacrolimus provides rapid and prolonged relief of the major symptoms of eczema (e.g. pruritus, erythema, oedema, induration/papulation, excoriations, lichenification and oozing or crusting). Tacrolimus was shown to be particularly effective in treating eczema of the head and neck. Moreover, other studies have demonstrated that skin atrophy is not induced with tacrolimus treatment. This represents an important advantage over traditional topical corticosteroid therapy, which can cause skin atrophy as a result of the inhibition of collagen synthesis. Consequently, topical corticosteroids must be used with caution in areas of thinner skin such as the face, neck and flexors, and when applied over longer periods of time. Tacrolimus is available in two strengths of ointment (0.1 and 0.03%) licensed for twice-daily treatment of atopic eczema in adults and children. The 0.03% dose is licensed to treat both children over 2 years and adults, whilst the higher dose is reserved for adults only.

Introduction

Treatment options available for atopic eczema are largely concerned with rehydrating the skin and relieving inflammation and pruritus. Topical corticosteroids are widely regarded as first-line therapy for atopic eczema, principally because of their potent anti-inflammatory effects. However, their use must be carefully monitored, particularly with prolonged use, as they can be associated with symptom rebound, tachyphylaxis (tolerance to therapy over time) and skin atrophy (or skin thinning). The occurrence of skin atrophy, in particular, makes corticosteroids an undesirable option for the treatment of facial eczema and for longer-term use, and this has been the main driving force behind the pursuit of alternative therapies for the condition.

Tacrolimus is a calcineurin inhibitor discovered in 1984 during a screening programme for naturally occurring immunosuppressants.[1] This compound was originally called FK506 and its potent T-cell inhibitory activity led to its worldwide adoption, along with ciclosporin, in the prevention of organ transplant rejection. The fact that oral ciclosporin had additional activity in improving the symptoms of psoriasis and atopic eczema, but was not active topically, provided the rationale for the development of topical formulations of tacrolimus, specifically designed to treat atopic eczema. Tacrolimus targets a variety of immune cells within the skin which are directly involved in the pathogenesis of atopic eczema, including epidermal dendritic cells, T cells, mast cells, basophils and keratinocytes.[1]

Tacrolimus is currently indicated for the treatment of moderate-to-severe atopic eczema unresponsive to conventional therapy, and should be prescribed by physicians experienced in treating the condition. Outside the UK, in Korea and Japan for example, tacrolimus is approved for the treatment of eczema of all severities. Tacrolimus is available in two ointment strengths. The 0.1% ointment is indicated for treatment of adults with atopic eczema whereas the 0.03% ointment is indicated for the treatment of children aged from 2 to 15 years and for adults. In addition to its use in atopic eczema, clinical evidence suggests that tacrolimus may also be useful in treating conditions such as psoriasis, pyoderma gangrenosum, lichen planus, graft-*versus*-host-disease, allergic contact dermatitis and steroid-induced rosacea. However, tacrolimus is not currently licensed for these alternative indications.[2]

Pharmacology

Chemistry

☞ *The chemistry of tacrolimus is of essentially academic interest and most healthcare professionals will, like you, skip this section.*

Structurally, tacrolimus is an 822 Da macrolide compound isolated from *Streptomyces tsukubaensis* (Figure 1). The structure shares commonality with other macrolide immunosuppressants including ascomycin, rapamicin and finally, pimecrolimus, which is its closest structural relative. Tacrolimus is a larger molecule than the classical topical corticosteroid used to treat atopic eczema, hydrocortisone (362 Da), but is still sufficiently small to allow it to be absorbed efficiently into the skin, in contrast with ciclosporin (1203 Da).

Figure 1. Chemical structure of tacrolimus (FK506).

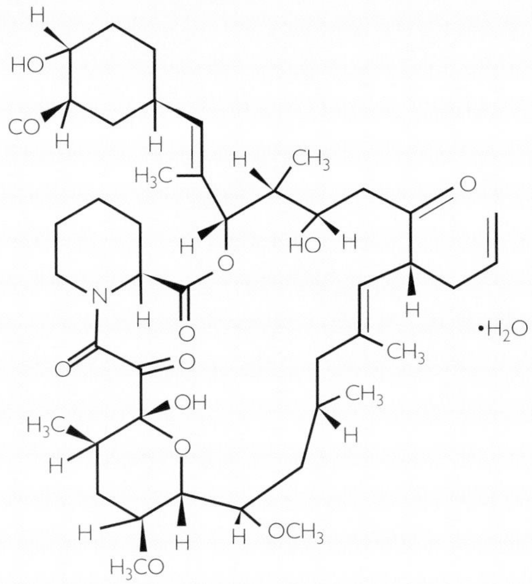

Mechanism of action

Inhibition of calcineurin

In common with other macrolide immunosuppressants, like pimecrolimus, tacrolimus inhibits the production of inflammatory cytokines by inhibiting calcineurin. Tacrolimus inhibits T-cell activation by binding to specific cytosolic proteins called immunophilins (Figure 2). Specifically, tacrolimus binds to the FK506-binding protein (FKBP)-12, or macrophilin-12, and this complex in turn binds to, and inactivates calcineurin (a cytosolic calcium- and calmodulin-dependent protein phosphatase). The inactivation of calcineurin means that it no longer performs its role of dephosphorylating cytosolic nuclear factors, which are thus unable to translocate into the nucleus where they would normally combine with their nuclear-localised binding partner and initiate RNA transcription of key cytokine mediators. Thus, an important secondary intracellular target of tacrolimus is the nuclear factor of activated T cells or NF-AT, which binds to the promoter region of specific genes and initiates transcription of interleukin 2 (IL-2), which in turn activates cytotoxic T cells, natural killer (NK) cells and B cells.[3] In the same way, tacrolimus is thought to inhibit the transcription of other cytokines, which also have key roles in the pathogenesis of atopic eczema, including IL-3, IL-4, IL-5, granulocyte-macrophage colony-stimulating factor (GM-CSF), interferon (IFN)-γ and tumour necrosis factor (TNF)-α.[3–5]

> In common with other macrolide immunosuppressants, tacrolimus inhibits the production of inflammatory cytokines by inhibiting calcineurin.

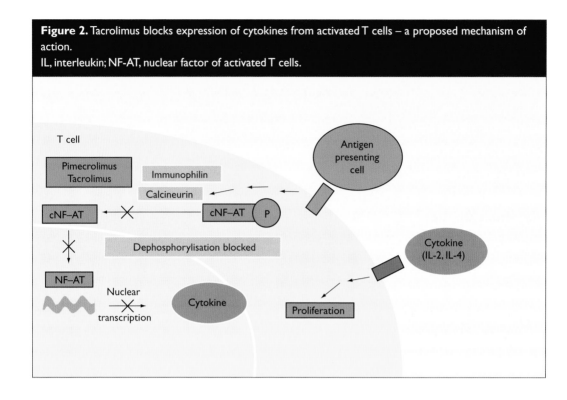

Figure 2. Tacrolimus blocks expression of cytokines from activated T cells – a proposed mechanism of action.
IL, interleukin; NF-AT, nuclear factor of activated T cells.

Other targets of tacrolimus

An additional target for tacrolimus is FcεR1, a high-affinity receptor for immunoglobulin E (IgE) present on antigen-presenting cells such as Langerhans cells, inflammatory dendritic epidermal cells (IDEC), macrophages, mast cells and basophils. The binding of IgE to this receptor triggers the release of inflammatory mediators including IL-12, IL-6, IL-8, TNF-α and monocyte chemoattractant protein (MCP)-1 via transcription factors such as NF-κB. Tacrolimus down-regulates FcεR1 expression on Langerhans cells and IDECs such that antigen presentation is decreased. Tacrolimus also inhibits the release of inflammatory mediators from mast cells and basophils, though it is not known whether this effect is mediated by down-regulation of FcεR1. It has also been suggested that the expression of FcεR1 may be mediated by NF-AT, but so far this remains largely speculative.[6]

Additional effects of tacrolimus, which may or may not be related to its immunomodulatory properties include:

- antifungal properties against *Malassezia furfur*
- inhibition of histamine and serotonin release from skin mast cells
- up-regulation of IL-10 receptors
- increased levels of p53 (a critical protein involved in the regulation of cell growth and apoptosis)
- inhibition of the expression of the IL-2 receptor (CD25) and the co-stimulatory molecules CD80 and CD40.[5,7]

Tacrolimus has no direct antimicrobial effect but has been shown to indirectly reduce populations of *Staphylococcus aureus* found on the skin.[8] Tacrolimus may also exert its immunomodulatory effects via enhanced expression of transforming growth factor (TGF)-β – a multifunctional cytokine with potent immunosuppressive activity which inhibits IL-2-dependent T- and B-cell proliferation and the production of TNF-α, TNF-β and IFN-γ.[3]

A summary of the role of these various immune cell types, their role in immunity and the effects of tacrolimus upon their activity is presented in Table 1.

Pharmacokinetics

Tacrolimus is administered topically since it has excellent epidermal absorption and demonstrates very little systemic uptake (Figure 3).[9–11] Typically, 5 g of tacrolimus, 0.1%, is used per day, which most closely

☞ *The pharmacokinetics of a drug are of interest to healthcare professionals because it is important for them to understand the action of a drug on the body over a period of time.*

Table 1. Cell types and inflammatory mediators of the immune response inhibited by tacrolimus.[2–4]

Skin cell type	Role in immunity	Effect of tacrolimus
T-helper cells	Production of IL-2, IL-3, IL-4, IL-5, IL-13, IFN-γ, GM-CSF, TNF-α, which are all involved in cytotoxic T-cell activation and proliferation	Reduces cytokine release via calcineurin inhibition
Langerhans cells	IgE-mediated antigen presentation and stimulation of T cells	Down-regulation of FcεRI, IL-2 and IL-8 receptors
IDECs	IgE-mediated antigen presentation and stimulation of T cells	Down-regulation of FcεRI resulting in decreased antigen presentation
Mast cells	Stem cell factor, IgE-induced degranulation (i.e. release of preformed inflammatory mediators from granules)	Blocks degranulation from cells and inhibits the release of histamine, cytokines and prostaglandin 2
Basophils	Release of histamine and other inflammatory mediators	Inhibits release of inflammatory mediators, possibly via FcεRI inhibition
Eosinophils	Recruited to produce reactive oxygen species, cytotoxic granules and inflammatory mediators	Role of tacrolimus so far unknown
Keratinocytes	Secrete IL-6, IL-7, IL-8, GM-CSF, chemokines and IL-10 receptor	Upregulates IL-10 receptor and may decrease the chemokine, RANTES. Inhibits T-cell induced keratinocyte apoptosis

GM-CSF, granulocyte-macrophage colony-stimulating factor; IDECs, inflammatory dendritic epidermal cells; IFN, interferon; IgE, immunoglobulin E; IL, interleukin; TNF, tumour necrosis factor.

Figure 3. Systemic absorption of tacrolimus after topical application.[11] Mean tacrolimus blood concentrations were measured after initial topical application of ointment to adult Japanese patients with atopic eczema (n=3)[9] or adult US (Caucasian) patients with atopic eczema (n=6).[10]

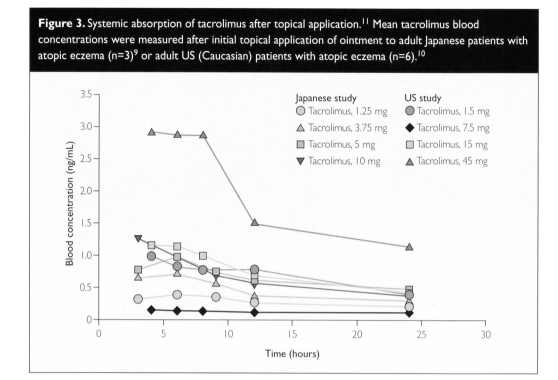

equates to the 5 mg daily dose of tacrolimus referred to in Figure 3.[12,13] In studies of varying duration – ranging from 3 weeks to 1 year – conducted in adults and children with moderate-to-severe atopic eczema, blood concentrations of tacrolimus were undetectable and below the limit of quantification (<0.5 ng/mL in two studies and 0.025 ng/mL in the other) in the majority of patients (75–90%).[12–15] For the purposes of comparison, it is worth noting that concentrations of tacrolimus administered orally to transplant patients who are likely to experience the most serious treatment-related side-effects, are up to 20 ng/mL. Increased toxicity is typically associated with systemic tacrolimus concentrations greater than 20 ng/mL, whilst systemic immunosuppressant effects may be expected at concentrations between 5 and 20 ng/mL.

Studies have shown that damaged skin absorbs tacrolimus at a seven-fold higher rate than intact skin, since healed skin regains percutaneous barrier function.[16] This presents a self-regulatory role, because as the skin heals, less drug is absorbed over the course of the treatment.[5]

The lack of systemic absorption is particularly important because calcineurin – the primary target of tacrolimus – is found throughout the body and is particularly abundant in the central nervous system and the kidney.

Given the minimal absorption of tacrolimus from the skin, the determination of the pharmacokinetic properties of the topical formulation of the drug is problematic. Therefore, these properties can only be determined accurately from dedicated studies which have examined the pharmacokinetics of tacrolimus when taken orally.

Preclinical studies

Safety and efficacy in animal models

For topically applied drugs, toxicity at the site of application and systemic toxicity secondary to skin absorption are both of potential concern and thus require extensive evaluation prior to embarking on human clinical studies. The skin of the Yucatan hairless micropig has similar absorptive properties to that of humans and therefore represents a useful model to evaluate the safety and efficacy of tacrolimus. Long-term safety evaluations of tacrolimus in this animal model revealed minimal systemic absorption of the drug after topical application. The systemic absorption after topical application is even lower in humans, as demonstrated by the pharmacokinetic studies described in the preceding section.[9–11] Studies performed *in vivo* and in animal models have indicated that when applied topically, tacrolimus acts locally via multiple cell types (i.e. T cells, mast cells, basophils and dendritic cells) and inhibits inflammatory skin reactions.[17] A recent investigation into the immunomodulatory effects of tacrolimus was performed in a mouse model of atopic eczema in which symptoms were induced upon exposure to mite antigen – a major environmental factor responsible for atopic eczema in humans (see Disease Overview).[18] On day 17 of treatment with tacrolimus, 0.03, 0.1 and 0.3%, thickening of the ears, erythema, oedema, scaling and excoriation were all reduced in treated animals compared with controls. Histopathological examination revealed decreased eosinophil infiltration and mast cell degranulation in lesions of mice treated with tacrolimus. Immunohistochemical analysis showed that CD4+ cells, IL-4 and IFN-γ were also reduced. Dermal expression of intercellular adhesion molecule (ICAM)-1, vascular cell adhesion molecule (VCAM)-1 and TNF-α were all reduced in the active treatment group compared with animals receiving placebo. This study also examined the effects of tacrolimus on eczema symptoms in the affected ear and demonstrated that the activity of tacrolimus was localised to the site of application.[18]

> Long-term safety evaluation of tacrolimus in this animal model revealed minimal systemic absorption of the drug after topical application.

Clinical efficacy

Preliminary clinical trials

Preliminary placebo-controlled trials demonstrated the potential of tacrolimus for the management of symptoms of atopic eczema. Primary symptoms of eczema which are monitored and targeted for improvement by any topical therapy should include the following:

- pruritus
- erythema
- oedema
- induration/papulation

- excoriations
- lichenification
- oozing/crusting.

The efficacy and tolerability of tacrolimus was evaluated in 213 patients, aged 13–60 years with moderate-to-severe atopic eczema, in a phase 2, randomised, double-blind, 3-week, multicentre study.[15] Three different doses of tacrolimus ointment (0.03, 0.1 and 0.3%) were compared with the ointment vehicle used as a control. The study investigators reported significantly greater improvements in the severity of primary symptoms (i.e. pruritus, oedema and erythema) and secondary symptoms (i.e. oozing/crusting, excoriation, lichenification and dryness of non-involved skin) of atopic eczema in patients treated with all three tacrolimus doses compared with those receiving the vehicle ointment. There were, however, no significant differences in efficacy reported between the three different doses of tacrolimus that were applied. The results of this phase 2 study are summarised in Table 2.[15]

The tacrolimus clinical development programme

An extensive programme of clinical trials (the largest ever conducted in dermatology) evaluating the efficacy and safety and tolerability of tacrolimus ointment in the treatment of atopic eczema began in the 1990s and included 12-week vehicle-controlled studies, short- and long-term comparative studies and several long-term safety studies, in children older than 2 years and in adults.[19] In general, the clinical development programme for tacrolimus has demonstrated that it offers rapid and effective long-term treatment of moderate-to-severe atopic eczema in both adults and children.

> Tacrolimus offers rapid and effective long-term treatment of moderate-to-severe atopic eczema in both adults and children.

Table 2. Median percentage decrease in symptom scores with tacrolimus (0.03–0.3%) and vehicle from baseline to the end of treatment (3 weeks).[15]

	Vehicle (n=54)	Tacrolimus dose[a] 0.03% (n=54)	0.1% (n=54)	0.3% (n=51)
Score 1				
Trunk and extremities	22.5	66.7[b]	83.3[b]	75.0[b]
Face and neck	25.0	71.4[b]	83.3[b]	83.3[b]
Score 2				
Trunk and extremities	21.8	61.5[b]	71.4[b]	70.0[b]
Face and neck	27.3	70.6[b]	75.0[b]	77.8[b]

Score 1 represents total body score of the severity of pruritus, oedema and erythema, whilst score 2 represents score 1 plus total scores for oozing or crusting, excoriation, lichenification and dryness of non-involved skin.
[a]tacrolimus applied twice daily.
[b]$p<0.001$ vs vehicle.

Methods of assessment

Clinical trials that evaluate new therapies for atopic eczema are reliant upon consistent and sensitive measures of changes in disease severity. Many efficacy parameters have been used to provide clinical assessment of atopic eczema. These include:

- physician's global evaluation of clinical response
- EASI (Eczema Area and Severity Index)
- mEASI (modified EASI)
- SCORAD (SCORing Atopic Dermatitis)
- SASSAD (Six Area, Six Sign Atopic Dermatitis)
- IGA (Investigators' Global Assessment)
- patients' assessment score
- assessment of severity of pruritis
- parents' index of quality of life.[13,20–23]

The physician's global evaluation of clinical response is widely employed in clinical studies that evaluate the efficacy of treatments for atopic eczema (Table 3).[13] Another of the most commonly used scoring indices employed is the EASI, which rates the severity of erythema, infiltration and/or papulation, excoriation and lichenification on a scale ranging from zero to three (where zero represents no symptoms and three represents severe symptoms), along with the percentage of body surface area affected by eczema in four body regions (head and neck, lower limbs, upper limbs and trunk). A recent modification of this scale, the mEASI, also incorporates a score for pruritis (a fundamental symptom of atopic eczema), rather than rating it separately as is performed in many other studies. The SCORAD is an alternative scoring system similar to the EASI which additionally evaluates dryness and oozing/crusts, pruritus and sleep loss. Other trials have employed variations on these themes or simply score individual symptoms.

Table 3. Rating scale for physician's global assessment of clinical response.[13]

Rating	Improvement (%)
Cleared	100
Excellent improvement	90–99
Marked improvement	75–89
Moderate improvement	50–74
Slight improvement	30–49
No appreciable improvement	0–29
Worse	<0

Short-term studies in adults and children

The efficacy of tacrolimus ointment, 0.03% and 0.1%, for the treatment of atopic eczema in adult patients was investigated in two 12-week randomised, double-blind studies conducted in 41 centres in the USA.[24] The study group (632 subjects, aged 15–79 years) were defined by diagnosis of atopic eczema of at least moderate severity and which covered 10–100% of body surface area. Of those randomised to receive tacrolimus, up to 75% completed the study compared with only 32% who received vehicle. The high drop-out rate of participants in the vehicle group was attributed to a lack of efficacy. The proportion of patients in whom disease improvement was at least 90% (excellent improvement or cleared as defined by the physician's global evaluation of clinical response [Table 3]) was significantly higher in those treated with tacrolimus, 0.03% (27.5 *vs* 6.6%; *p*<0.001), and in those treated with tacrolimus, 0.1% (36.8 *vs* 6.6%; *p*<0.001), compared with vehicle. The higher dose of tacrolimus was also shown to confer a greater success rate than the 0.03% dose (*p*<0.05). In terms of symptom scores, as evaluated by the EASI, tacrolimus treatment conferred significantly greater improvements compared with vehicle and the improvement was again greater with the 0.1% dose than with the 0.03% dose (Figure 4).[24] The improvement in symptoms was observed as early as 1 week after the start of tacrolimus treatment. Furthermore, pruritus (as assessed by patients) was dramatically improved by tacrolimus treatment, although no differences were reported between the two dosages in this regard.

> Tacrolimus treatment conferred significantly greater improvements compared with vehicle and the improvement was again greater with the 0.1% dose than with the 0.03% dose.

Figure 4. Improvement in total clinical scores and the Eczema Area and Severity Index (EASI) with tacrolimus, 0.03 and 0.1%, compared with vehicle in adult patients with at least moderately severe atopic eczema.[24]

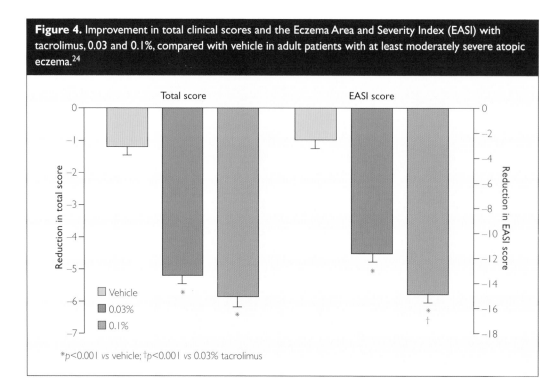

*p<0.001 vs vehicle; †p<0.001 vs 0.03% tacrolimus

The short-term efficacy of tacrolimus has also been evaluated in two paediatric studies: one a 3-week study in children aged 7–16 years (n=180); the other a 12-week study in children aged 2–15 years (n=351).[13,25] Patients enrolled in both studies had moderate-to-severe disease at baseline, affecting 5–30% of body surface area in the 7–16 year age group and 10–100% of body surface area in the 2–15 year age group. In the 3-week study, the mean percentage improvement on the mEASI was greater in all three tacrolimus treatment groups (0.03, 0.1 and 0.3%) compared with vehicle ($p<0.001$).[25] It should be noted, however, that this was a phase 2 dose-ranging study and tacrolimus is not licensed for use at doses higher than 0.1%. Differences between the tacrolimus and vehicle groups reached statistical significance by day 8 of treatment. Clinical efficacy in the head and neck region was also specifically evaluated in this study and revealed a beneficial effect of tacrolimus treatment compared with the control. Thus, symptom scores improved by 65, 83 and 81% in the tacrolimus, 0.03, 0.1 and 0.3%, treatment groups, whilst scores deteriorated by 2% in the vehicle group (all active treatment groups $p<0.001$ vs vehicle). No serious systemic adverse events were apparent over the course of this study. The most common side-effects were pruritus and skin burning at the site of application, which occurred predominantly during the first 4 days of treatment. However, such events were reported with similar frequency in both the vehicle group and active treatment groups.

Similarly, in the 12-week study, both the 0.1% and 0.03% doses of tacrolimus were shown to be significantly more effective than vehicle with regard to all efficacy endpoints, with no differences between the two doses reported.[13] Efficacy measures in this study included physician's global evaluation, patient–parent assessment, EASI score (Figure 5), total symptom scores, percentage body surface area affected and patients' assessment of pruritus. Moreover, equal efficacy and tolerability of tacrolimus was reported in younger (2–6 years) and older (7–15 years) children.

In both the 3- and the 12-week studies, no increase in adverse events was apparent with higher doses of topical tacrolimus.[13,25] Present preliminary data from two retrospective studies of 49 infants in total, suggest that tacrolimus may be well tolerated and provide effective relief of the symptoms of moderate-to-severe eczema in this age group.[26,27]

Long-term studies in adults and children

The aforementioned short-term studies have indicated that tacrolimus is effective and well tolerated in the treatment of atopic eczema in both adults and children. However, since atopic eczema is often chronic and relapsing there is also a need to evaluate the long-term efficacy and tolerability of tacrolimus.

An open-label, non-comparative study has been performed across 30 European centres, over a period of 6 months to 1 year, in adults (aged 18–70 years with moderate-to-severe atopic eczema affecting 5–60% of body surface area) receiving tacrolimus, 0.1%.[14] Tacrolimus was shown

> Equal efficacy and tolerability of tacrolimus was reported in younger (2–6 years) and older (7–15 years) children.

Figure 5. Improvement in total clinical scores and the Eczema Area and Severity Index (EASI) with tacrolimus, 0.03 and 0.1%, compared with vehicle in paediatric patients (aged 2–15 years) with moderate-to-severe atopic eczema.[13]

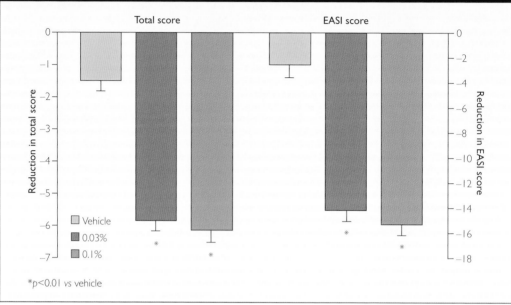

*p<0.01 vs vehicle

Long-term use of tacrolimus was also associated with decreases in affected body surface area and ointment use over the 12-month course of the study.

to be effective in improving the symptoms of atopic eczema (as measured by the mEASI). In common with the short-term studies, the improvement in symptoms was rapid and was apparent during the first week of treatment, and was sustained thereafter with maximal improvement appearing to plateau by the third month. The long-term use of tacrolimus was also associated with decreases in affected body surface area and ointment use over the 12-month course of the study. Moreover, the investigator's assessment of global improvement showed that as the study progressed, an increasing proportion of patients began to experience 90–100% improvement in symptoms (Figure 6).[14]

The effectiveness of tacrolimus in preventing disease flares (defined as disease status requiring topical corticosteroid therapy for at least 3 days) has not yet been fully addressed prospectively, but preliminary data, employing retrospective analyses of data from the aforementioned study, indicate that treatment with tacrolimus, 0.1%, prevented progression to disease flares in 89.7% of adult patients.[28]

An open-label, long-term, non-comparative safety study was performed over 1 year in children, aged 2–15 years with moderate-to-severe atopic eczema, across 31 centres in the USA.[29] Efficacy was evaluated by assessment of per cent body surface area affected, EASI score and assessment of pruritus, whilst safety was determined by incidence of adverse events and plasma measures of hepatic and renal function, electrolytes, glucose and total IgE. After 1 week of therapy, improvement was reported in all efficacy variables, and most patients

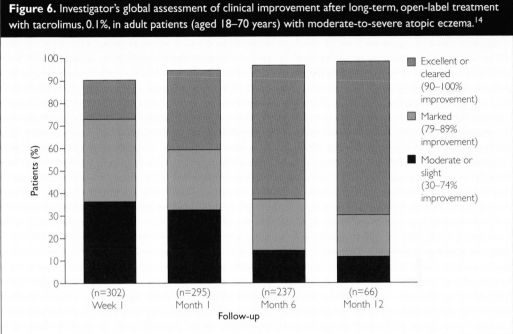

Figure 6. Investigator's global assessment of clinical improvement after long-term, open-label treatment with tacrolimus, 0.1%, in adult patients (aged 18–70 years) with moderate-to-severe atopic eczema.[14]

continued to improve over the 12-month treatment period. Of the 255 patients enrolled in the study, 61 were deemed to be completely clear of atopic eczema by the investigator and treatment was discontinued. The median time to treatment discontinuation was 92 days. However, 40 of these children experienced an investigator-documented recurrence of atopic eczema after a median of 36 days. Given that there is no current cure for atopic eczema and that relapses are to be expected after treatment withdrawal, this is not necessarily a surprising observation. The most common adverse events reported were localised skin burning and pruritus on application, but these reactions generally resolved over time (Figure 7). Other adverse events reported included skin infections and non-application site events such as influenza-like symptoms, headache, fever, asthma, allergic reactions and cough. However, these events did not alter over the course of treatment, and appeared to be seasonal in the case of influenza-like symptoms, and were considered not to be related to the drug treatment.

Further preliminary data from two large, open-label, non-comparative multicentre studies, conducted over 2–4 years (the first comprising over 7900 patients and the second almost 800 patients with moderate-to-severe atopic eczema) have further demonstrated the continuing long-term efficacy of tacrolimus, 0.1%, in both children and adults.[30,31] These studies await full publication in the medical literature.

Figure 7. The occurrence of pruritus and skin burning over time after tacrolimus, 0.1%, application in children aged 2–15 years.[1,29]

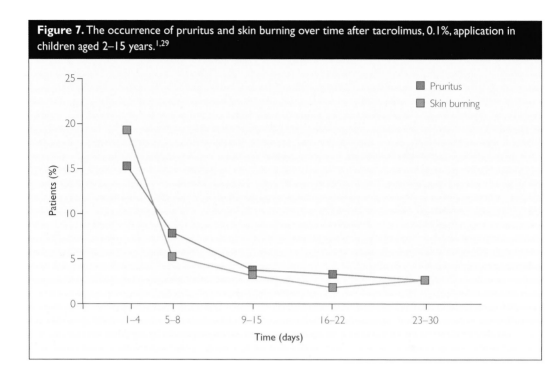

Comparative studies in adults and children

Comparison with topical corticosteroid therapy

Two large phase 3 studies were designed to compare the safety and efficacy of tacrolimus, 0.1 and 0.03%, with topical corticosteroid treatment in adults aged 16–70 years and in children aged 2–15 years, with moderate-to-severe atopic eczema.[21,32] The topical corticosteroid treatment chosen for the adult study was hydrocortisone butyrate ointment, 0.1%, which is a widely prescribed medium potent-to-potent corticosteroid, whilst the comparator in the paediatric study was hydrocortisone acetate ointment, 1%, a mild and commonly prescribed corticosteroid widely used for the treatment of atopic eczema in children.

A total of 570 adults and 560 children, recruited from 27 European centres, were randomised to receive one of the four therapies over a 3-week period. The mEASI was the primary endpoint employed in both studies to evaluate clinical efficacy. An improvement in symptoms was apparent 3 days after starting treatment in all groups in both studies and was maintained until treatment completion at the third week (Table 4).

In the paediatric study, all of the efficacy parameters evaluated demonstrated that tacrolimus, 0.1 and 0.03%, offered superior efficacy compared with hydrocortisone acetate, 1%. This was true of the per cent affected body surface area, mEASI and the physician's global evaluation of clinical response measures (Table 4).[21,32]

The performance of tacrolimus in the adult study showed that both body surface area affected and the efficacy measures detailed in Table 4

Table 4. Efficacy outcomes in adults (16–70 years) and children (2–15 years) treated with tacrolimus or corticosteroid therapies applied over 3 weeks.[21,32]

	Children (n=560)			Adults (n=570)		
	HCA	Tacrolimus		HCB	Tacrolimus	
	1%	0.03%	0.1%	0.1%	0.03%	0.1%
Median decrease from baseline in mEASI (area under the curve [%])						
Whole treated area	36.0	55.2[a]	60.2[a,b]	63.9	53.0[c]	63.5
Head and neck	43.3	62.5[a]	75.2[a,b]	"same response as main analysis"		
Physician's global evaluation of clinical response (% of patients)						
Excellent	15.7	38.5[a]	48.4[a]	51.4	37.6[d]	49.2
Marked	32.4	62.6	73.9	70.5	58.2	76.5
Moderate	51.4	80.2	85.3	79.2	79.9	85.0

[a]$p<0.001$ vs HCA
[b]$p<0.01$ vs tacrolimus, 0.03%
[c]$p<0.001$ vs HCB or tacrolimus, 0.1%
[d]$p<0.05$ vs HCB or tacrolimus, 0.1%
HCA, hydrocortisone acetate; HCB, hydrocortisone butyrate.

were equally improved by both tacrolimus, 0.1%, and hydrocortisone butyrate, 0.1%. However, tacrolimus, 0.03%, offered significantly less efficacy in this adult patient population than either the 0.1% doses of tacrolimus or hydrocortisone butyrate.

Overall, these data indicate that tacrolimus ointment, 0.1%, has comparable efficacy to hydrocortisone butyrate, 0.1%, when treating adults with atopic eczema, and is superior to hydrocortisone acetate, 1%, in managing atopic eczema in children. Thus, tacrolimus offers an effective and acceptable alternative to topical corticosteroids for patients with moderate-to-severe atopic eczema.[21,33]

> Tacrolimus offers an effective and acceptable alternative to topical corticosteroids for patients with moderate-to-severe atopic eczema.

Frequency of application

The current licensed dose of tacrolimus for children with moderate-to-severe atopic eczema is a twice-daily application of the 0.03% ointment. However, a recent study set out to determine the potential for once-daily tacrolimus treatment regimen compared with twice-daily treatment in this patient group.[34] Children aged between 2 and 15 years were randomised to three treatment groups in this double-blind, 3-week long study: hydrocortisone acetate, 1% twice daily; tacrolimus, 0.03% once daily; tacrolimus, 0.03% twice daily. Twice-daily application of tacrolimus was found to be more effective than once-daily application in improving symptoms of eczema (decrease in mEASI from baseline: 78.7 vs 70%; $p=0.007$), whilst both applications of tacrolimus were more effective than hydrocortisone, 1% (decrease in mEASI from baseline: 47.2%; both $p<0.001$).

A subgroup analysis of these data reported that patients with severe atopic eczema at baseline responded significantly better to twice-daily application than once-daily treatment (decrease in mEASI from baseline: 75.5 *vs* 54.1%; *p*=0.001). In contrast, patients with moderate disease at baseline responded equally well to both treatment regimens (81.6 *vs* 79.3%; no *p*-value reported).[34]

In terms of safety data taken from these comparative studies, skin burning and pruritus were the only adverse events to show a higher incidence in adults treated with tacrolimus compared with corticosteroid treatment (*p*<0.05). However, in children only skin burning was more prevalent with tacrolimus treatment compared with hydrocortisone acetate, though this symptom was generally mild and transient and did not lead to discontinuation from the study. There did not appear to be a difference in the incidence of adverse events amongst children receiving either once- or twice-daily tacrolimus. The most common adverse events that occurred in this paediatric study are summarised in Table 5.[34]

Comparison with pimecrolimus

Current UK guidelines recommend the use of tacrolimus for moderate-to-severe atopic eczema, in children aged over 2 years at a 0.03% dosage and in adults aged over 16 years at a 0.1% dose, whilst pimecrolimus, 1%, is indicated for treatment of mild-to-moderate atopic eczema in patients over 2 years. A recent study has, for the first time, performed a direct analysis of the two agents over a 6-week period.[35] This study

Table 5. Incidence of the most common adverse events occurring in children treated for 3 weeks with tacrolimus (0.03%, once or twice daily) or hydrocortisone acetate (1%, twice daily).[33]

Adverse event	Incidence of adverse event (n [%])		
	Hydrocortisone acetate (1%) (n=207)	Tacrolimus (0.03%) Once daily (n=207)	Twice daily (n=210)
Skin burning	30 (14.5)	48 (23.2)	50 (23.8)
Pruritus	33 (15.9)	38 (18.4)	45 (21.4)
Folliculitis	8 (3.9)	8 (3.9)	11 (5.2)
Influenza syndrome	11 (5.3)	6 (2.9)	12 (5.7)
Skin erythema	2 (1.0)	6 (2.9)	6 (2.9)
Fever	4 (1.9)	5 (2.4)	6 (2.9)
Headache	6 (2.9)	2 (1.0)	8 (3.8)
Rash	2 (1.0)	3 (1.4)	6 (2.9)
Skin infection	6 (2.9)	3 (1.4)	6 (2.9)
Pustular rash	5 (2.4)	3 (1.4)	3 (1.4)

reported results from three separate patients cohorts: children (aged 2–15 years) with mild disease (n=425); children (aged 2–15 years) with moderate-to-severe disease (n=225); adults (aged over 16 years) with disease ranging from mild to very severe (n=413). Treatment was with tacrolimus, 0.03%, in children with mild disease, and tacrolimus, 0.1%, in the other two groups, with pimecrolimus, 1%, the comparator in all cases.

Combined analysis of all three groups demonstrated a greater proportion of pimecrolimus-treated patients withdrawing from the study due to lack of efficacy (35/533) compared with tacrolimus-treated (13/530; $p<0.01$). Moreover, greater improvements in EASI scores were reported after 6 weeks' treatment with tacrolimus compared with pimecrolimus (52.8 vs 39.1%; $p<0.0001$). These observations, together with other data indicating superiority of tacrolimus over pimecrolimus in terms of reducing pruritus, percentage body surface area affected and success as determined by the investigators' global assessment, support current guidelines for the use of tacrolimus in moderate and severe disease.

This study has provided some important and unique information on the management of mild atopic eczema in paediatric patients. In this patient cohort, a greater number of patients from the pimecrolimus group withdrew as a consequence of adverse events than those in the tacrolimus group (4.6 vs 0%, respectively; $p<0.01$). Moreover, in terms of efficacy, tacrolimus proved more effective than pimecrolimus after 1 week of treatment in terms of reducing the EASI (39.2 vs 31.2%; $p<0.05$), per cent body surface area affected (41.0 vs 32.9%; $p<0.05$) and itch ($p<0.05$). Whilst there was a trend for superiority of tacrolimus over pimecrolimus in these parameters at the end of the study, only the reduction in itch remained significantly improved by tacrolimus compared with pimecrolimus after the 6-week treatment period. These data indicate that tacrolimus, 0.03%, appears to be at least as effective as pimecrolimus, 1%, in the treatment of mild paediatric atopic eczema. However, more clinical trial data will be necessary to determine which of the two therapies consistently has the better tolerability and efficacy profile in this patient population.

Comparison with oral ciclosporin

A small study (n=30) of 6 weeks' duration was conducted to compare the efficacy of topical tacrolimus ointment, 0.1% twice daily, with oral ciclosporin (3 mg/kg, once daily) in patients with moderate-to-severe atopic eczema.[22] Response to treatment was assessed using the SCORAD system. This study demonstrated that tacrolimus conferred significantly greater improvements in symptoms of atopic eczema than ciclosporin, with significant differences between the two treatment groups apparent from 14 to 35 days after treatment with the greatest difference between the treatments observed after 28 days of therapy (tacrolimus 24.8±1.1 vs ciclosporin 43.5±0.4; $p<0.001$). However, by the end of treatment (day 42), SCORAD scores were virtually identical in both groups (tacrolimus 7.3 and ciclosporin 8.6). Tacrolimus conferred a greater reduction in the symptoms of pruritus, erythema and sleep loss, compared with oral ciclosporin. No differences in serum total IgE was observed over the treatment period in either group.[22]

Combination therapy

A combination approach to treatment has the potential to increase the efficacy of therapy whilst reducing the frequency of adverse events. This was recently addressed in a small study (n=57; patients aged 16–65 years with atopic eczema affecting 5–20% of body surface area), which investigated whether the efficacy of tacrolimus used concomitantly with the topical corticosteroid, clocortolone pivalate,[a] was more effective than tacrolimus monotherapy.[36] In terms of improvements in the dermatological sum score and symptoms of excoriation, induration and erythema, the combination therapy was more effective than tacrolimus alone. The combination therapy also resulted in lower scores for the occurrence of burning and pruritus at the site of application. Therefore, such an approach may be especially useful in those patients particularly prone to these unpleasant side-effects.

> The combination of tacrolimus and topical steroid therapy appears to be an effective strategy for the treatment of facial and whole body eczema.

A further Japanese study retrospectively examined clinical data from patients who had been receiving daily treatment with either tacrolimus and/or topical corticosteroid therapy for at least 6 months.[37] The authors of this analysis reported that the reduction in the dose of topical corticosteroid resulting from the concomitant application of tacrolimus, attenuated the incidence and the severity of corticosteroid-induced adverse events including hypertrichosis, telangiectasia and skin atrophy. This study also reported that combination therapy reduced the number of patients with intractable atopic eczema. Consequently, from the currently available data, it would appear reasonable to conclude that the combination of tacrolimus and topical steroid therapy appears to be an effective strategy for the treatment of facial and whole body eczema.

Efficacy for facial application

The head, neck and flexures are therapeutically challenging areas as the skin is thinner in these regions and is also more prone to irritation. These limitations, combined with the association of traditional corticosteroid therapy with skin atrophy, hypopigmentation, secondary infections and acne has presented significant challenges to physicians when managing atopic eczema in these problem areas.[38,39]

> A greater overall response to treatment was reported in the head and neck areas compared with other regions treated.

Initial data demonstrating the promising efficacy of tacrolimus in treating refractory facial eczematous lesions was confirmed in a combined analysis of three double-blind randomised studies, which showed that tacrolimus was effective in treating atopic eczema in the head and neck area in both adults and children.[39,40] Symptoms of erythema, oedema, excoriation, oozing and scaling were all significantly improved with the tacrolimus, 0.1%, regimen compared with the lower

---

[a]Clocortolone pivalate is not available in the UK.

dose (0.03%). Moreover, a greater overall response to treatment was reported in the head and neck areas compared with other regions treated. In addition, the incidence of adverse events remained similar for the head and neck regions compared with other treated body surfaces.[39]

The occurrence of skin thinning caused by decreased collagen synthesis is a recognised limitation of the long-term use of topical corticosteroids for treating skin diseases such as atopic eczema. To date, tacrolimus has not been associated with skin atrophy in any clinical trials that have been reported. However, to confirm this, the incidence of skin atrophy was directly assessed in a year-long, open-label trial, which compared two groups of patients with atopic eczema – one receiving conventional therapy (mostly corticosteroids of intermediate potency) and tacrolimus, 0.1% twice daily – with an untreated control group of healthy volunteers.[41] Collagen synthesis and skin thickness (evaluated by ultrasound) were determined at baseline. Tacrolimus treatment over 1 year was not associated with any skin thinning or atrophy. Specifically, in the tacrolimus group, the synthesis of procollagen propeptide types I and III increased by 65 and 158 µg/L ($p<0.001$), respectively, over the course of the study. This contrasted with conventional corticosteroid therapy which resulted in non-significant reductions in procollagen propeptide type I (11.5 µg/L) and type III (21.5 µg/L). Furthermore, skin thickness in those treated with tacrolimus increased by 114.7 µm over the 12-month period, whilst the conventional therapy group exhibited a decrease in skin thickness of 110.7 µm ($p<0.001$ tacrolimus *vs* conventional therapy). Although it is fair to conclude that tacrolimus appears to be free from the detrimental skin atrophogenic effects of corticosteroid therapy, the increase in collagen synthesis and concurrent increase in skin thickness may not be directly attributable to tacrolimus therapy. Baseline levels of procollagen were significantly lower in the group randomised to receive tacrolimus than in healthy volunteers, which presumably was a consequence of prior corticosteroid therapy. Therefore, increases in procollagen levels in the tacrolimus group may be more reflective of return to healthy baseline levels, in the absence of corticosteroid treatment, rather than a direct mechanistic feature of tacrolimus therapy. In addition, the measures of skin thickness employed in this study must also be interpreted with caution since there are clear associations of atopic eczema with inflammation and oedema. These symptoms may represent confounding factors in such assessments of skin thickness.

> Tacrolimus treatment over 1 year was not associated with any skin thinning or atrophy.

Efficacy in special patient populations – racial variation

African–American sufferers of atopic eczema treated with low-dose tacrolimus for 12 weeks, showed no improvement in symptoms (as assessed by the physician's global evaluation of clinical response) with tacrolimus, 0.03%, compared with control. However, tacrolimus, 0.1%, provided significant benefit (defined as 90–100% improvement) compared with vehicle (29 *vs* 7%; $p=0.002$).[24] This was not an unexpected finding since decreased transcutaneous penetration of chemicals and drugs has been reported in African–American skin such that we might expect a higher dose to be necessary to achieve clinical benefit.[42] In a combined analysis of data from three short-term trials with tacrolimus, 0.03 and 0.1%, the incidence of adverse events appeared to be similar in black or white skin.[3]

The efficacy of tacrolimus has also been assessed in two studies examining Korean and Taiwanese populations – both conducted over 4 weeks – in those suffering from moderate-to-severe eczema, which affected at least 10% of the body surface area.[43,44] The smaller of these studies examined Taiwanese children (n=26, aged 2–15 years) and adults (n=42, aged ≥16 years), who were treated with tacrolimus, 0.03 or 0.1% respectively.[44] Greater than moderate improvement (≥50%) was observed in over 80% of both children and adults whilst the per cent body surface area affected decreased by 47% in children and by 34% in adults ($p<0.001$). The EASI score was also significantly reduced by tacrolimus treatment in both children (58%) and adults (50%, $p<0.001$).[44]

The Korean study examined the effect of tacrolimus, 0.03%, in adults and children (n=180, aged 2–57 years) and reported good efficacy both in terms of EASI (8.0±9.1 at week 4 *vs* 19.7±12.9 at baseline; $p<0.05$) and the investigator's global assessment, where moderate improvement was seen over the 4-week period (3.99±1.24 at week 4 *vs* 4.54±1.15 at week 1; $p<0.05$).[43] The most common adverse event reported in both patient populations was burning and itching at the site of application, but this was most severe a few hours after application and declined in severity thereafter. These studies indicate that tacrolimus represents a well tolerated and effective treatment when managing moderate-to-severe atopic eczema in Taiwanese and Korean populations.

Safety and tolerability

As reported in this review, the most common adverse events attributed to tacrolimus therapy are associated with local irritation at the site of application – most commonly skin burning (including a burning sensation, pain, stinging and soreness), pruritus and erythema. The majority of clinical studies report that the burning sensation and pruritus are experienced more frequently in patients with severe or extensive disease but, importantly, these symptoms resolve during the first few days of therapy.[5] Influenza-like symptoms, headache, folliculitis, sinusitis, skin rash, alcohol intolerance, acne, skin tingling, hyperaesthesia, back pain, myalgia and cyst formation have also been reported less frequently after tacrolimus use.[5] In six patch-test studies in healthy volunteers, single or repeated exposure to tacrolimus ointment, 0.03–0.3%, was compared with vehicle, other products on the market (i.e. hydrocortisone or betamethasone valerate) and a known irritant as positive control. These studies reported that, relative to these other products, tacrolimus was not inherently irritating, sensitising, phototoxic or photoallergenic when applied to intact skin.[11]

The long-term (1 year) safety of tacrolimus has also been examined in clinical trials and the most common adverse events associated with tacrolimus treatment are detailed in Figure 8.[14] These data again confirm that the majority of adverse events occur at the site of application. In an open-label, 1-year study where tacrolimus, 0.1%, was applied twice daily, no significant increases in adverse events were observed. As seen in other studies, the incidence of the most common side-effect – skin burning – actually decreased over time (days 1–4: 45.3%; months 10–12: 2.1%; Figure 7). Furthermore, tacrolimus was shown not to accumulate in the blood with repeated long-term application.[5,14] Laboratory assessments of hepatic and renal function, serum electrolytes and serum IgE, were also performed and were all found to be unaffected by tacrolimus application.[5]

A similar investigation was performed in children aged 2–15 years.[32] Again, of the few adverse events noted, skin burning and itching at the application site were the most commonly reported. These episodes were usually short in duration (under 10 minutes for burning and under 1 hour for itching) and usually subsided after a few days of continuing treatment. The most common non-application site events were influenza-like symptoms, headache and fever, although the vast majority of these were not considered to be related to tacrolimus ointment.

> In an open-label, 1-year study where tacrolimus, 0.1%, was applied twice daily, no significant increases in adverse events were observed.

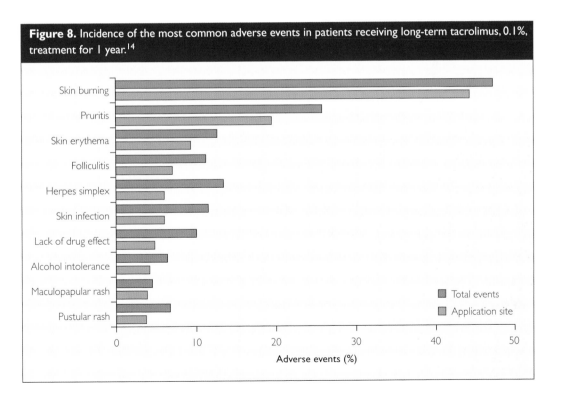

Figure 8. Incidence of the most common adverse events in patients receiving long-term tacrolimus, 0.1%, treatment for 1 year.[14]

Carcinogenic potential

In order to determine whether topical tacrolimus was associated with any carcinogenic effects, a 2-year study was conducted in mice with five different ointment concentrations of tacrolimus (0.03–3.0%).[45] No increase in the incidence of skin tumours was observed, although there was a statistically significant increase in the incidence of pleiomorphic and undifferentiated lymphoma associated with the highest dose of tacrolimus. However, the clinical relevance of this latter observation is questionable given that this dose is considerably higher than the maximum dose licensed for use in humans. These effects were not observed with either the 0.03 or 0.1% doses of tacrolimus and indeed, in mice, antitumour-promoting effects of tacrolimus have been documented.[46] However, given that up to 45% of patients undergoing organ transplantation who receive systemic immunosuppression develop skin cancer within 10 years, caution is advised.[47] Although the currently available data does not indicate a link between the long-term topical use of tacrolimus and an increased incidence of skin cancer, the avoidance of UV-light therapy and minimal exposure to the sun is recommended by the manufacturer.[45,47]

Contraindications

Tacrolimus should not be used by patients with hypersensitivity to macrolides in general, or to tacrolimus or any of the excipients. Patients with Netherton's syndrome are advised not to use tacrolimus due to the potential for increased systemic absorption.[5] Tacrolimus can also cross the placental membrane and is excreted in human milk. Therefore, tacrolimus ointment should not be used by pregnant women, whilst breast-feeding during tacrolimus treatment is also not recommended.[5]

Association with infection

Atopic eczema is associated with bacterial and viral skin infections and since tacrolimus acts by modulating the immune system, there is a theoretical potential for an increase in the incidence of infection.[37] Bacterial infection with *S. aureus* is a common and sometimes serious complication of atopic eczema and may cause skin lesions such as impetigo or scalded skin syndrome. This bacterium is found on lesional skin of more than 90% of patients with atopic eczema but is present on the skin of less than 10% of healthy subjects.[19] The use of tacrolimus has been associated with an early decrease in the number of *S. aureus* colonies in skin lesions as they heal. A review of data from five clinical trials (including both short- and long-term studies in both children and adults) examined the correlation between tacrolimus treatment and the risk of skin infection and concluded that treatment with either, tacrolimus ointment, 0.03 or 0.1%, did not increase the risk of cutaneous bacterial, viral or fungal infections in patients with atopic eczema.[6,12–14,24,29] However, tacrolimus applied at either concentration was associated with an increased incidence of folliculitis in adults but not in children.[6]

Treatment with either 0.03 or 0.1% tacrolimus ointment did not increase the risk of cutaneous bacterial, viral or fungal infections in patients with atopic eczema.

Similar theoretical concerns have also been raised regarding the effects of tacrolimus on the immune status of children post-vaccination. However, a small pilot study found no effect of tacrolimus on the immune status of children following pneumococcal vaccination.[48]

Impact on quality of life and patient preference

The available evidence clearly points to the fact that tacrolimus is an effective therapeutic option for the treatment of atopic eczema. Given its efficacy, tacrolimus also has the potential to improve the impaired quality of life associated with this condition.

Consequently, the effects of tacrolimus therapy upon the quality of life of both children and adults were evaluated in a 12-week, randomised double-blind study.[49] Markers of quality of life evaluated in this study included effects on routine daily and leisure activities, productivity at work or at school, social interactions, self-consciousness and quality of sleep. An improved quality of life was reported in adults receiving tacrolimus therapy at both doses, compared with vehicle, and a greater improvement in quality of life from baseline was observed in the 0.1% tacrolimus group compared with the 0.03% group. In children, there was no difference between the two ointment strengths but both the 0.1 and 0.03% doses resulted in improved quality of life compared with vehicle treatment.[49] Patient preference for continuation of allocated therapy was also surveyed by this study. Among adults, 79.7% of the 0.1% tacrolimus group and 68.8% of the 0.03% tacrolimus group reported that they 'would continue or very likely would continue' with the study drug they had received. Only 28.8% of the vehicle-treated group reported that they would be 'very likely to continue' with their allocated (vehicle) treatment. A similar questionnaire was completed by parents of children (5–15 years) and toddlers (2–4 years) receiving the same 12-week therapies. In this case, more than 80% of parents of both toddlers and children in both the 0.1 and 0.03% tacrolimus groups reported that they 'would continue or very likely would continue' with the study drug their child had received. This compared with 50 and 39.5% of parents of children and toddlers, respectively, in the vehicle-treated groups, who reported that they would continue with the (vehicle) treatment allocated. Only 3.3 and 2.2% of parents of children and toddlers, respectively, who received tacrolimus, 0.1%, reported that they 'would not continue or very unlikely would continue' with the allocated therapy.

> More than 80% of parents of both toddlers and children reported that they 'would continue or very likely would continue' with tacrolimus.

Pharmacoeconomics

Despite the clear benefits of tacrolimus treatment, few studies have examined its relative cost-effectiveness as a treatment for atopic eczema, a disease estimated to result in an annual UK expenditure of £465 million (at 1996 prices).[50] One US-based study compared the cost-effectiveness of high-potency topical corticosteroids with tacrolimus, for the treatment of moderate-to-severe atopic eczema in patients not responsive to, or poorly controlled with, mid-potency topical corticosteroids.[51] This analysis focused on prescription drug charges and physician costs over the course of 1 year and assumed that the same quantity of ointment was used in both treatment groups. The principal conclusion of this analysis was that tacrolimus ointment was a more cost-effective option over a 2-week treatment period, but both tacrolimus and corticosteroids had similar cost-effectiveness over a 4-week therapy cycle. Although tacrolimus ointment is more expensive than the majority of topical corticosteroids on a weight-for-weight basis, patients receiving tacrolimus in this study spent less time in secondary therapy, which may contribute to the greater cost-effectiveness of tacrolimus reported. In addition, as yet unpublished data – derived from a UK-focused economic modelling comparison of corticosteroid use compared with tacrolimus therapy – indicates that tacrolimus is a more cost-effective option than corticosteroids in adults with either moderate or severe eczema, although the average cost per person in children (aged 2–16 years) was slightly higher for tacrolimus than for corticosteroid treatment.[52] An additional pharmacoeconomic analysis has been conducted to determine the relative cost-effectiveness ratios (using prescription drug costs from 2002) of tacrolimus and pimecrolimus when managing patients with moderate atopic eczema who did not respond to, or were not well-controlled with, topical corticosteroids.[53] Given the absence of direct head-to-head clinical trial data at the time that this analysis was conducted, treatment outcomes were based on EASI scores from relevant clinical trials. Using this approach, it was estimated that, in this patient population, pimecrolimus was approximately 60% as effective as tacrolimus over a 2–4-week treatment period. On the basis of these data, average cost-effectiveness ratios were calculated at US$7.34 and US$11.34 per disease controlled day, for tacrolimus and pimecrolimus, respectively. Furthermore, sensitivity analyses revealed that pimecrolimus would be more cost-effective only if it were 90% as effective as tacrolimus. However, it is essential that these data are substantiated using data from prospectively conducted, head-to-head clinical trials of both agents before any firm conclusions can be drawn.

Despite the strong clinical evidence for the use of agents such as tacrolimus to treat a wide variety of patient populations with atopic eczema, recent guidelines drawn up by the National Institute for Clinical Excellence (NICE) in the UK do not currently recommend tacrolimus, or indeed pimecrolimus, as first-line treatments for atopic eczema of any severity.[54] Overall, their health economic assessments concluded that tacrolimus was estimated to be more costly than topical corticosteroids alone, with the exception of its use as a second-line treatment of body eczema in adults. Therefore, at present, according to the NICE guidelines, tacrolimus therapy is considered as a second-line option in the treatment of moderate-to severe atopic eczema in adults and children (older than 2 years) who have not responded to prior topical corticosteroid therapy or where there is significant risk of important adverse events from the continued use of topical corticosteroids (i.e. irreversible skin atrophy).

Key points

- Tacrolimus is recommended for the treatment of atopic eczema in both children (older than 2 years) and adults.

- Tacrolimus acts via the inhibition of calcineurin to reduce the production of inflammatory cytokines, which are implicated in the pathogenesis of atopic eczema.

- Tacrolimus begins to reduce symptoms of atopic eczema within the first week of use, with improvements in symptoms continuing over a year of continued application.

- Continuous treatment with tacrolimus over 1 year leads to a decrease in affected body surface area and a reduction in the amount of ointment used.

- Studies have shown that tacrolimus, 0.1%, offers comparable efficacy to hydrocortisone butyrate in adults with atopic eczema. Moreover, tacrolimus has superior efficacy when compared with hydrocortisone acetate in children with the condition.

- Unlike topical corticosteroid therapy, tacrolimus does not cause skin atrophy and therefore represents a valuable alternative therapeutic agent, particularly when treating affected areas with thinner skin such as the head and neck.

- Tacrolimus is not absorbed systemically to any significant degree following topical application of tacrolimus.

- The most common side-effects associated with tacrolimus treatment are skin burning and itching at site of application, but these adverse effects are usually short-lived and resolve within 1 week of treatment initiation.

References

A list of the published evidence which has been reviewed in compiling the preceding section of *BESTMEDICINE.*

1 Rico MJ, Lawrence I. Tacrolimus ointment for the treatment of atopic dermatitis: clinical and pharmacologic effects. *Allergy Asthma Proc* 2002; **23**: 191–7.

2 Nghiem P, Pearson G, Langley RG. Tacrolimus and pimecrolimus: from clever prokaryotes to inhibiting calcineurin and treating atopic dermatitis. *J Am Acad Dermatol* 2002; **46**: 228–41.

3 Cheer SM, Plosker GL. Tacrolimus ointment. A review of its therapeutic potential as a topical therapy in atopic dermatitis. *Am J Clin Dermatol* 2001; **2**: 389–406.

4 Mrowietz U. Macrolide immunosuppressants. *Eur J Dermatol* 1999; **9**: 346–51.

5 Gupta AK, Adamiak A, Chow M. Tacrolimus: a review of its use for the management of dermatoses. *J Eur Acad Dermatol Venereol* 2002; **16**: 100–14.

6 Fleischer AB, Ling M, Eichenfield L *et al.* Tacrolimus ointment for the treatment of atopic dermatitis is not associated with an increase in cutaneous infections. *J Am Acad Dermatol* 2002; **47**: 562–70.

7 Panhans-Gross A, Novak N, Kraft S, Bieber T. Human epidermal Langerhans' cells are targets for the immunosuppressive macrolide tacrolimus (FK506). *J Allergy Clin Immunol* 2001; **107**: 345–52.

8 Pournaras CC, Lubbe J, Saurat JH. Staphylococcal colonization in atopic dermatitis treatment with topical tacrolimus (Fk506). *J Invest Dermatol* 2001; **116**: 480–1.

9 Kawashima M, Nakagawa H, Ohtsuki M, Tamaki K, Ishibashi Y. Tacrolimus concentrations in blood during topical treatment of atopic dermatitis. *Lancet* 1996; **348**: 1240–1.

10 Alaiti S, Kang S, Fiedler VC *et al.* Tacrolimus (FK506) ointment for atopic dermatitis: a phase I study in adults and children. *J Am Acad Dermatol* 1998; **38**: 69–76.

11 Bekersky I, Fitzsimmons W, Tanase A *et al.* Nonclinical and early clinical development of tacrolimus ointment for the treatment of atopic dermatitis. *J Am Acad Dermatol* 2001; **44**: S17–27.

12 Soter NA, Fleischer AB, Webster GF, Monroe E, Lawrence I. Tacrolimus ointment for the treatment of atopic dermatitis in adult patients: part II, safety. *J Am Acad Dermatol* 2001; **44**: S39–46.

13 Paller A, Eichenfield LF, Leung DY, Stewart D, Appell M. A 12-week study of tacrolimus ointment for the treatment of atopic dermatitis in pediatric patients. *J Am Acad Dermatol* 2001; **44**: S47–57.

14 Reitamo S, Wollenberg A, Schopf E *et al.* Safety and efficacy of 1 year of tacrolimus ointment monotherapy in adults with atopic dermatitis. The European Tacrolimus Ointment Study Group. *Arch Dermatol* 2000; **136**: 999–1006.

15 Ruzicka T, Bieber T, Schopf E *et al.* A short-term trial of tacrolimus ointment for atopic dermatitis. European Tacrolimus Multicenter Atopic Dermatitis Study Group. *N Engl J Med* 1997; **337**: 816–21.

16 Russell JJ. Topical tacrolimus: a new therapy for atopic dermatitis. *Am Fam Physician* 2002; **66**: 1899–902.

17 Bekersky I, Lilja H, Lawrence I. Tacrolimus pharmacology and nonclinical studies: from FK506 to protopic. *Semin Cutan Med Surg* 2001; **20**: 226–32.

18 Sasakawa T, Higashi Y, Sakuma S *et al.* Topical application of FK506 (tacrolimus) ointment inhibits mite antigen-induced dermatitis by local action in NC/Nga mice. *Int Arch Allergy Immunol* 2004; **133**: 55–63.

19 Kapp A, Allen BR, Reitamo S. Atopic dermatitis management with tacrolimus ointment (Protopic). *J Dermatolog Treat* 2003; **14**: 5–16.

20 Hanifin JM, Thurston M, Omoto M *et al.* The eczema area and severity index (EASI): assessment of reliability in atopic dermatitis. EASI Evaluator Group. *Exp Dermatol* 2001; **10**: 11–8.

21 Reitamo S, Rustin M, Ruzicka T *et al.* Efficacy and safety of tacrolimus ointment compared with that of hydrocortisone butyrate ointment in adult patients with atopic dermatitis. *J Allergy Clin Immunol* 2002; **109**: 547–55.

22 Pacor ML, Di Lorenzo G, Martinelli N *et al.* Comparing tacrolimus ointment and oral cyclosporine in adult patients affected by atopic dermatitis: a randomized study. *Clin Exp Allergy* 2004; **34**: 639–45.

23 Berth-Jones J. Six area, six sign atopic dermatitis (SASSAD) severity score: a simple system for monitoring disease activity in atopic dermatitis. *Br J Dermatol* 1996; **135(Suppl 48)**: 25–30.

24 Hanifin JM, Ling MR, Langley R, Breneman D, Rafal E. Tacrolimus ointment for the treatment of atopic dermatitis in adult patients: part I, efficacy. *J Am Acad Dermatol* 2001; **44**: S28–38.

25 Boguniewicz M, Fiedler VC, Raimer S *et al.* A randomized, vehicle-controlled trial of tacrolimus ointment for treatment of atopic dermatitis in children. Pediatric Tacrolimus Study Group. *J Allergy Clin Immunol* 1998; **102**: 637–44.

26 Housman TS, Norton AB, Feldman SR *et al.* Tacrolimus ointment: utilization patterns in children under age 2 years. *Dermatol Online J* 2004; **10**: 2.

27 Patel RR, Vander Straten MR, Korman NJ. The safety and efficacy of tacrolimus therapy in patients younger than 2 years with atopic dermatitis. *Arch Dermatol* 2003; **139**: 1184–6.

28 Remitz A, Petan J. Flare prevention with long-term use of 0.1% tacrolimus ointment in children and adults with atopic dermatitis. 12th Congress of the European Academy of Dermatology and Venereology. Barcelona, Spain, 2003.

29 Kang S, Lucky AW, Pariser D, Lawrence I, Hanifin JM. Long-term safety and efficacy of tacrolimus ointment for the treatment of atopic dermatitis in children. *J Am Acad Dermatol* 2001; **44**: S58–64.

30 Paller A, Hanifin J, Eichenfield L, Clark R, Rico MJ. *Tacrolimus ointment monotherapy is a safe and effective treatment for atopic dermatitis long-term (more than 3 years).* American Academy of Dermatology. San Francisco, 2003.

31 Koo JMH, Prose N, Fleischer A, Rico MJ. Safety and efficacy of tacrolimus ointment monotherapy in over 7900 atopic dermatitis patients: results of an open-label study. 20th World Congress of Dermatology. Paris, France, 2002.

32 Reitamo S, Van Leent EJ, Ho V *et al.* Efficacy and safety of tacrolimus ointment compared with that of hydrocortisone acetate ointment in children with atopic dermatitis. *J Allergy Clin Immunol* 2002; **109**: 539–46.

33 Reitamo, S. *0.1% tacrolimus ointment is significantly more efficacious than a steroid regimen in adults with moderate-to-severe atopic dermatitis.* The European Academy of Dermatology and Venereology. Budapest, Hungary, 2004.

34 Reitamo S, Harper J, Bos JD *et al.* 0.03% Tacrolimus ointment applied once or twice daily is more efficacious than 1% hydrocortisone acetate in children with moderate to severe atopic dermatitis: results of a randomized double-blind controlled trial. *Br J Dermatol* 2004; **150**: 554–62.

35 Paller A, Lebwohl M, Fleischer A *et al.* Tacrolimus ointment is more effective than pimecrolimus cream with a similar safety profile in the treatment of atopic dermatitis: results from three randomized, comparative studies. *J Am Acad Dermatol* 2004; **52**: 810–22.

36 Torok HM, Maas-Irslinger R, Slayton RM. Clocortolone pivalate cream 0.1% used concomitantly with tacrolimus ointment 0.1% in atopic dermatitis. *Cutis* 2003; **72**: 161–6.

37 Furue M, Terao H, Moroi Y *et al.* Dosage and adverse effects of topical tacrolimus and steroids in daily management of atopic dermatitis. *J Dermatol* 2004; **31**: 277–83.

38 Reitamo S, Rissanen J, Remitz A *et al.* Tacrolimus ointment does not affect collagen synthesis: results of a single-center randomized trial. *J Invest Dermatol* 1998; **111**: 396–8.

39 Kang S, Paller A, Soter N *et al.* Safe treatment of head/neck AD with tacrolimus ointment. *J Dermatolog Treat* 2003; **14**: 86–94.

40 Kawakami T, Soma Y, Morita E *et al.* Safe and effective treatment of refractory facial lesions in atopic dermatitis using topical tacrolimus following corticosteroid discontinuation. *Dermatology* 2001; **203**: 32–7.

41 Kyllonen H, Remitz A, Mandelin JM, Elg P, Reitamo S. Effects of 1-year intermittent treatment with topical tacrolimus monotherapy on skin collagen synthesis in patients with atopic dermatitis. *Br J Dermatol* 2004; **150**: 1174–81.

42 Berardesca E, Maibach H. Racial differences in skin pathophysiology. *J Am Acad Dermatol* 1996; **34**: 667–72.

43 Won CH, Seo PG, Park YM *et al.* A multicenter trial of the efficacy and safety of 0.03% tacrolimus ointment for atopic dermatitis in Korea. *J Dermatolog Treat* 2004; **15**: 30–4.

44 Lan CC, Huang CC, Chen YT *et al.* Tacrolimus ointment for the treatment of atopic dermatitis: report of first clinical experience in Taiwan. *Kaohsiung J Med Sci* 2003; **19**: 296–304.

45 Fujisawa Ltd. Protopic® (tacrolimus) ointment 0.03% and 0.1%. *Summary of product characteristics.* Japan, 2004.

46 Jiang H, Yamamoto S, Nishikawa K, Kato R. Anti-tumor-promoting action of FK506, a potent immunosuppressive agent. *Carcinogenesis* 1993; **14**: 67–71.

47 Thestrup-Pedersen K. Tacrolimus treatment of atopic eczema/dermatitis syndrome. *Curr Opin Allergy Clin Immunol* 2003; **3**: 359–62.

48 Rico MJ, Stiehm ER, Roberts RL *et al.* Tacrolimus ointment does not suppress the immune system of children aged 2–12. 12th Congress of the European Academy of Dermatology and Venereology. Barcelona, Spain, 2003.

49 Drake L, Prendergast M, Maher R *et al.* The impact of tacrolimus ointment on health-related quality of life of adult and pediatric patients with atopic dermatitis. *J Am Acad Dermatol* 2001; **44**: S65–72.

50 Herd RM, Tidman MJ, Prescott RJ, Hunter JA. The cost of atopic eczema. *Br J Dermatol* 1996; **135**: 20–3.

51 Ellis CN, Drake LA, Prendergast MM *et al.* Cost-effectiveness analysis of tacrolimus ointment versus high-potency topical corticosteroids in adults with moderate to severe atopic dermatitis. *J Am Acad Dermatol* 2003; **48**: 553–63.

52 Rustin M. *Cost-effectiveness of tacrolimus ointment in the treatment of adults and children with moderate to severe atopic dermatitis in the UK.* The European Academy of Dermatology and Venereology. Budapest, Hungary, 2004.

53 Abramovits W, Boguniecqicz M, Prendergast MM, Tokar M, Tong KB. Comparisons of efficacy and cost-effectiveness of topical immunomodulators in the management of atopic dermatitis. *J Med Econ* 2003; **6**: 1–14.

54 National Institute for Clinical Excellence. *Tacrolimus and pimecrolimus for atopic eczema.* Technology Appraisal 82, August 2004. *www.nice.org.uk*

Acknowledgements

Figure 3 is adapted from Bekersky *et al.*, 2001.[11]
Figure 4 is adapted from Hanifin *et al.*, 2001.[24]
Figure 5 is adapted from Paller *et al.*, 2001.[13]
Figure 6 is adapted from Reitamo *et al.*, 2000.[14]
Figure 7 is adapted from Rico and Lawrence, 2002.[1]
Figure 8 is adapted from Reitamo *et al.*, 2000.[14]

PATIENT NOTES
Dr Tim Mitchell

Drug development in atopic eczema

On the face of it, it would be reasonable to question the fact that this book concentrates on just two of the most recently licensed drugs. To understand why this is the case, it is worth looking briefly at some history.

Over 50 years ago, a revolution took place in the management of many skin diseases, including atopic eczema, when topical steroids were introduced. These treatments were clean and easy to use creams and ointments, which rapidly reduced inflammation and brought the condition under control. They were so much better than, and soon replaced, messy, smelly agents such as tar which did work but left many people wondering if the 'cure' was any better than the eczema itself. Consequently, it was not surprising that the topical steroids took off so quickly and soon became established as first-line treatments for different severities of eczema and for different parts of the body. As the first steroid preparations were quite potent, side-effects were soon apparent, and the most obvious of these was skin thinning. This provided the impetus to develop less potent steroids specifically for use on vulnerable areas of the body such as the face and skin creases (flexures). However, the introduction of these less potent steroids did not happen quickly enough to prevent steroids developing a reputation for causing problems, and many patients, and indeed doctors, became wary of using them at all. This wariness was extreme enough in some cases to be labelled 'steroid phobia' and some patients, or parents in the case of children, refused to use any steroids.

Topical steroids took off quickly and soon became established as first-line treatments for different severities of eczema and for different parts of the body.

What are the potential problems with topical corticosteroids?

- Loss of collagen in the deeper layers of the skin. Collagen has an important structural role giving strength and support to other structures. Loss of collagen leads to thinning of the skin, stretch marks, easy tearing and bruising.
- Dampening down of the local immune system resulting in susceptibility to infection. Steroids have a more generalised effect in the skin rather than specifically dealing with inflammation.
- Tachyphylaxis – a loss of effect with continued use, which can lead to the need for more potent steroids.
- Triggering of other types of rashes (usually on the face) including visible capillaries giving a red appearance, and acne-like spots around the cheeks and mouth.

• Adverse effects on the rest of the body. If too much cream is applied over too large an area of the skin, enough can be absorbed to cause the same sort of problems seen with steroids taken by mouth. These so-called systemic effects include weight gain, growth problems and an increased propensity towards the development of diabetes.

All of these problems can be avoided if steroids are used correctly, at the right strength and for the right length of time. This latter point really means that they are meant as short-term treatments only, with various guidelines suggesting a maximum of 2 weeks treatment in most cases.

It is surprising, therefore, that whilst alternative types of treatment are clearly welcome it has taken more than 50 years for anything other than subtle modifications of existing steroids to reach the market.

One barrier to the development of new treatments is the cost of developing and bringing a new product to the market, particularly with the current need to prove safety or at the very least to show the risk of any problems developing (see Reader's Guide). This associated cost will mean that new products will be far more expensive than steroids which, as would be expected for 50-year-old products, are often only a matter of a few pence.

Since the topical steroids were first introduced we have seen vast changes in many other areas of medicine, with very expensive drugs gaining widespread acceptance in important areas such as heart disease, diabetes and asthma. The difference with eczema is in the perception of the 'importance' of the illness and the willingness to invest at a national level. Atopic eczema doesn't normally kill people but it does makes their lives miserable!

The calcineurin inhibitors – tacrolimus and pimecrolimus

The two new drugs, pimecrolimus and tacrolimus, are very welcome additions to the range of treatments currently available for atopic eczema. Their names are not all that easy to pronounce, but a look at tacrolimus shows how its name came about. It is derived from a fungus that grows on the slopes of Mount **T**sukuba in Japan and is part of a class of compounds called ma**croli**des. This class of drugs includes some commonly used antibiotics such as erythromycin. The action of the drug is as an i**mmuno**suppressant, and so the name was coined. Tacrolimus has been around for longer than pimecrolimus and was first used to prevent organ rejection in transplant cases.

The preceding sections of this book examine the action of these drugs within the skin in detail. Like the steroids, tacrolimus and pimecrolimus act to reduce inflammation in the skin, but with a much more focused mechanism of action. As a

Like the steroids, tacrolimus and pimecrolimus act to reduce inflammation in the skin, but with a much more focused mechanism of action.

consequence, there is less potential for side-effects especially from loss of collagen and thinning of the skin. This allows them to be used on more delicate areas of the skin (such as the face and flexures) and for longer periods with less risk than the topical steroids. Nothing is, however, that simple. Any drug with beneficial effects also has the potential for some unwelcome or damaging side-effects. Modern drug development and testing goes a long way towards identifying these potential side-effects, at least in the short term. However, nobody would suggest that everything is known about possible side-effects from intermittent use over what could be many years or even decades with a chronic disease such as atopic eczema.

The indications for the two drugs vary, as can be seen from the licences granted to allow their prescribing. Pimecrolimus is considered to be 'milder' and suitable for use in the short-term treatment of mild-to-moderate eczema and for intermittent long-term use to prevent the progression of episodes of increased itching and redness into definite eczema. Pimecrolimus is only available in one strength and should not be used for children under the age of 2 years. Tacrolimus has a different indication with the additional recommendation that it should only be used by doctors with experience in treating atopic eczema. It is suitable for use in treating moderate-to-severe atopic eczema where conventional treatments have failed or cannot be used. This may be because of previous side-effects with other treatments. Tacrolimus comes in two strengths – 0.03% for children aged 2–15 years and 0.1% for adults. Neither drug is licensed for use in children under 2 years of age, which is a pity because many of them will suffer from atopic eczema affecting areas of skin which are particularly sensitive to the adverse effects of topical steroids. The licences are given on the basis that the drugs work and do not have serious side-effects. As with most other drugs, however, there are some associated side-effects, but these are usually short term and in the form of skin irritation or a burning sensation.

Can we expect another revolution in the treatment of atopic eczema?

It will take some time for pimecrolimus and tacrolimus to find their place in the routine management of atopic eczema. They will not suit every patient but are very useful for patients who have had problems using topical steroids, whether this is established or anticipatory. Pimecrolimus is indicated for the prevention of flare progression but has not yet been tested against the occasional use of mild steroids for this indication. Therefore, further research is needed before its use is widened. Tacrolimus has been shown to be as effective as potent steroids, but since these do not tend to cause irritation and do not cause skin thinning if properly used, the price difference remains a valid reason to keep it in reserve.

Pimecrolimus and tacrolimus are very useful for patients who have had problems using topical steroids.

Despite these issues, it is very important that these drugs become more widely used and that enough 'expert patients' become familiar with them and work out their own ways of making the most of these new drugs. Many drugs end up being used outside the limits of their original licences once doctors and patients have become familiar with them. This is already happening with these new drugs. For example, dermatologists are using pimecrolimus on children under 2 years of age and the stronger 0.1% formulation of tacrolimus is also being used in some children. Patients given a tube of either cream may not follow the exact instructions given and use the creams intermittently or in combination with topical steroids. If this method proves successful, doctors must acknowledge the patients' expertise in managing their own skin condition and work with it. The idea of combining new treatments with existing ones has been very successful with other skin conditions such as psoriasis and could prove to be very successful in atopic eczema. For example, the steroid could act to reduce the local irritation associated with the newer drugs whilst, in turn, pimecrolimus and tacrolimus would reduce the amount of steroid used and, therefore, the potential for associated side-effects.

Future developments

It is far too early to judge these new drugs. They have been welcomed by many patients as a new type of treatment, free from the worst side-effects of steroids and will establish themselves as part of the overall management of atopic eczema in a way that might differ from their original licences. Moreover, if they are successfully established, this will encourage pharmaceutical companies to continue to research new varieties of calcineurin inhibitors in an attempt to minimise the chance of local irritation whilst maximising their beneficial effects. Competition will tend to drive down prices which should make the budget holders less wary of these new treatments.

The idea of combining new treatments with existing ones has been very successful with other skin conditions and could prove to be very successful in atopic eczema.

5. Improving practice

Dr Stephen Kownacki MB BS MRCGP
GP, Wellingborough, Northamptonshire
Hospital Practitioner in Dermatology, Northampton General Hospital Trust
Chairman, Primary Care Dermatology Society

Summary

Atopic eczema has a profound impact on the health and quality of life of individual patients and their families, with disease severity directly influencing the extent of this impairment. The condition also imposes a major burden on healthcare resource consumption and its associated costs. For example, in the primary care setting alone we can expect one patient in every 20 that we see to have atopic eczema. An appreciation and understanding of the burden of this major condition is essential if we are to motivate ourselves and our healthcare colleagues to find ways to manage it effectively. By examining how we currently deal with the problem of atopic eczema, we can identify areas where we can improve practice which will allow us to formulate effective management plans to ensure better care for our patients in the future. The involvement of the entire primary care team and the adoption of an education and awareness campaign for all practice staff will also help us manage the condition more effectively. As with any chronic condition, people living with eczema and their families are likely to benefit from an improved understanding of their condition. Support is widely available from a variety of different sources to assist in this. Effective diagnosis, of course, lies at the heart of successful clinical management, and whilst this is relatively straightforward for atopic eczema, there are a number of complicating factors including disease severity, which can ultimately affect treatment choice. Indeed, given that more severe disease presentation is associated with a more profound impact upon psychosocial factors, greater benefits for both the patient and their family can be attained when such patients are treated effectively. Lifestyle changes can help to

☞ *Remember that the author of the* Improving Practice *is addressing his healthcare professional colleagues rather than the 'lay' reader. This provides a fascinating insight into many of the challenges faced by doctors in the day-to-day practice of medicine (see Reader's Guide).*

minimise disease flares and improve the overall control of the condition and as we have seen in the preceding sections, a variety of pharmacological approaches are available to manage atopic eczema of varying severities. The recent introduction of the calcineurin inhibitors may lead to a paradigm shift in the way we manage acute exacerbations of atopic eczema, towards more effective prophylaxis in the longer-term.

Introduction

We have seen in the earlier sections of this edition of *BESTMEDICINE* that atopic eczema is a significant and growing problem for healthcare services, resulting in substantial direct costs to the health service and indirect costs to the individual and the broader economy. More importantly, atopic eczema profoundly impacts upon the quality of life and the general health of the individual patient and their family. Over recent years, we have seen a three-fold increase in the prevalence of atopic eczema, and in the developed world up to 20% of all children are likely to develop the condition. From these data, we can predict that in an average UK primary care practice each GP will see one dermatological problem for every six or seven consultations and, of these, about one-third will be cases of atopic eczema. This equates to approximately one patient presenting during each surgery.

> Atopic eczema profoundly impacts upon the quality of life and the general health of the individual patient and their family.

The majority of patients with atopic eczema are managed effectively in primary care using a multifaceted approach that includes the identification and avoidance of triggering factors for exacerbations, good skin care and the use of appropriate anti-inflammatory and antibiotic treatments where necessary. Referral to secondary care is only usually necessary in severe cases and where the patient has not responded adequately to treatment. Given the exceptionally high demand from patients for services to manage atopic eczema, it is essential that primary care professionals establish strategies to cope. It is no longer an option to remain ignorant or dismissive of such a major disease even if our medical schools still relegate dermatology to a minor section of education!

> It is no longer an option to remain ignorant or dismissive of such a major disease.

Management not just treatment

Like so many diseases managed in primary care, atopic eczema should be regarded as a management problem rather than a simple treatment choice. Knowing what to write on a prescription is only a very small part of the overall process. So what other factors do we need to consider, and are there special circumstances that make atopic eczema different from the other chronic diseases with which we have to deal?

Organisation

In the UK, in contrast to other chronic conditions such as asthma, dermatology has not been awarded special funding status. However, it is vital to remember that atopic eczema is a number one priority for those of our patients who suffer from this distressing condition. Therefore, I think it is critical that we carefully consider our approach to the management of our patients with atopic eczema. Important factors include:

- how do we interact with our patients when they first present?
- can patients get access to the right person easily and in an appropriate time frame?
- does your practice have a partner, health visitor or, if you are particularly lucky, a specialist nurse with dermatology expertise?
- are your reception/telephone/prescription staff sympathetic to signs of itch and distress, as well as the more dramatic disease presentations?

A prompt repeat prescription, perhaps asked for at an early stage, or a new antibiotic prescribed for a secondary infection may prevent family disruption, missed school days or even avoid a hospital admission. For this reason, I would strongly recommend awareness education for all the practice staff to complement the specific expertise within the nursing team along the same lines as asthma management.

> I would strongly recommend awareness education for all the practice staff to complement the specific expertise within the nursing team.

Equipment

Fortunately this section is mercifully small. There is, however, a need for good light, warm and private surroundings in which to examine the undressed patient (as the whole body needs to be assessed) and perhaps a magnifying glass for us older practitioners! The facility to take swabs for bacteria and viruses and to take mycological scrapings to exclude alternative or co-existent fungal disease is also required (e.g. a scalpel blade and some coloured paper or a universal specimen pot for nail clippings). A bath in which to soak a child before wet wrapping is a luxury that is only rarely needed, and probably leads us into the realms of intermediate or secondary care.

I find it very useful to have a selection of emollients in sample sizes, both of bath additives and topical applications, which can be sampled by patients and/or their carers. It is clear that the best emollient for any patient is the one that the patient favours and cannot be dictated by experts or by prescribing advisers. Here in the UK, the Skin Care Campaign (*www.skincarecampaign.org*) recently fought an attempted imposition of aqueous cream as the only permitted emollient. Whilst it may be a useful soap substitute, it contains far too much water and has a significant allergenic potential as well. It is vital that a choice of emollient is made available to our patients, particularly when we consider that there are many different skin types requiring different levels of grease; for example, black skin often requires more greasy applications.

> I find it very useful to have a selection of emollients in sample sizes, both of bath additives and topical applications, which can be sampled by patients and/or their carers.

Assessment

Effective and accurate diagnosis is a prerequisite for the successful management of any disease and although in the case of atopic eczema, it is usually straightforward, the consequences of mistakes can be distressing for the patient and embarrassing for the doctor! Despite this, there are some complicating factors in reaching an accurate diagnosis, which may affect ultimate treatment choice, including differential diagnosis and variations in the severity of disease presentation.

Other forms of eczema that should be considered when establishing a diagnosis include:

- discoid eczema which requires a higher potency corticosteroid and is more resistant to treatment
- allergic or contact eczema which may require patch testing and allergen avoidance
- asteototic eczema in the elderly where one should avoid potent steroids on the thinned and cracked skin
- varicose eczema often with auto-sensitisation to the trunk and upper limbs which will not settle until the primary lower leg eczema is effectively treated.

Seborrheic dermatitis in the infant may also confuse the diagnosis. However, unlike atopic eczema, it is not itchy and often involves the scalp (cradle cap) and the nappy area. It is likely to settle with the minimum of treatment using emollients and perhaps a weak corticosteroid. Remember, 'if it does not itch, it is not eczema'. But also be alert to scabies, since we can all miss it sometimes!

> Remember, 'if it does not itch, it is not eczema'.

A typical assessment and management plan may include the features outlined below.

- Record the age, type of onset, extent and severity of the disease, evidence of infection or lichenification, exacerbating factors, previous treatment prescribed to date and the patient's or carer's view of the success, or otherwise, of the treatment.
- Listen to the fears and sometimes the misunderstandings of disease and its treatments (e.g. equating steroids with bodybuilder anabolics). The degree of distress of the patient will also affect your approach. For example, more severe presentations of the disease will be associated with even greater distress and an appropriate and empathetic response is necessary, as is the selection of an appropriate therapeutic regimen.
- Offer empathy and education to the patient relating to the disease and its management, discuss alternative treatments and give advice as to 'what to do and when'.
- Provide written information using leaflets or booklets, but also, for example, personally tailored body maps. Also alert your patient to other sources of support and information. For example, in the UK, the National Eczema Society (*www.eczema.org*) is a useful source of such information and has many leaflets of its own which are very useful and can reinforce the advice that you give.

- Patient follow-up is vital to fine-tune and adjust treatment according to response. In particular, it also allows you to show your continued support or better still the support of the whole primary care team. Advice as to how and when patients should seek urgent help and from whom is also important.

Impact on quality of life

We should never underestimate the impact that any disease exerts on the quality of life of the patient and their family. It has been well documented that atopic eczema affects the psychosocial well-being of everyone that it touches. For example, the relentless itching associated with the disease can affect the individual's capacity for sleep and, in turn, can greatly affect their performance at school or work. Unsightly lesions can cause great distress to the patient, particularly in children, which can lead to their withdrawal from enjoyable activities and subsequent social isolation, and even retard social development in the more severe cases. The care of an affected child can also cause considerable stress and tension within a family, possibly leading to tension between spouses and siblings. Taken together, it is apparent that we should no longer regard atopic eczema as merely a minor skin disorder, but as a condition which can be a major handicap, with consequences for both the family and the community.

The degree of impairment in quality of life increases with increasing disease severity, with moderate-to-severe atopic eczema exacting a particularly profound effect on quality of life. For example, a recent Australian study has ranked the family stress related to the care of a child with moderate-to-severe atopic eczema as being significantly greater than that of the care of children with type 1 diabetes mellitus. As a consequence, effective management of moderate-to-severe disease offers real value in not only managing the physical symptoms of the disease but also the associated psychosocial distress.

> We should no longer regard atopic eczema as merely a minor skin disorder, but as a condition which can be a major handicap, with consequences for both the family and the community.

Lifestyle modification

Atopic eczema is a chronic relapsing incurable disease, which has inevitably attracted many misconceptions, often as a consequence of the failure of traditional medicine to manage the condition effectively. This has been further compounded by the fact that research has not yet taught us everything we need to know about the disease. An excellent illustration of this confusion is the example of breast-feeding, which was previously thought to have been protective in atopic eczema. However, a recent study has indicated that this may not be the case and indeed the effect may be the opposite! One of the latest suggestions with positive evidence is the ingestion of probiotics during the latter stages of pregnancy in order to reduce the likelihood of atopic eczema in the new infant. Despite this imperfection in our knowledge, we should not let it prevent us sharing what we have learnt from clinical studies or from our own clinical experience as long as we are clear as to where this comes from.

Avoidance of irritants and allergens is of major benefit and may preclude certain occupations such as nursing or hairdressing, where contact with chemicals is inevitable. As such, early career advice may save later disappointment. Dust-mite allergy is common and avoidance is difficult but worth trying if the eczema is particularly severe. Simple advice regarding soft toys, furnishings and carpets along with wet dusting and washing of pillows may be helpful but can be very complex and time consuming! Pets, especially cats, are a common allergen and their dander can persist for many years after the cat has gone. In addition, children can still be exposed to dander from their cat-owning school friends. However, once a cat is installed in a family home the emotional distress caused by its removal may actually outweigh any potential benefits of reduced exposure to animal dander. Indeed, stress is an identifiable factor in the development of eczema flares, which of course is easier to spot than cure, and can be both a cause and a consequence of a flare. Food additives and allergens provoke significant debate and are often one of the major reasons for referral into secondary care. In the very young (under 1 year of age) dietary measures (particularly cow's milk exclusion) have a much greater chance of helping atopic eczema. However, great care must be taken to ensure an adequate intake of nutrients, and thus professional dietary advice is strongly recommended. In older children and adults, the benefits are much less obvious unless of course the cause is clear (e.g. a sudden flare of the face after eating tomatoes). Avoiding the colourings in foodstuffs may also be worth trying and may not be so disruptive as the avoidance of a major foodstuff. Again, professional dietary advice might help the patient to achieve this.

In real life, however, the majority of patients' conditions are controlled by fairly simple and relatively safe treatment regimens, which preclude the need for significant changes in family life that major dietary manipulation requires. The availability of a broad therapeutic arsenal, which covers the range of disease severities that are likely to present in clinical practice means that patients' suffering can be minimised. Indeed, it is clear that the best benefit–effort ratios are achieved by those with more severe disease presentations.

Clinical management

Patients usually present in an acute flare situation looking for relief. However, before prescribing any treatment it is important to establish the cause of the flare. In my experience, the most common causes are increased scratching due to irritants such as raised environmental temperature, clothing, stress and/or concurrent skin infection. Infection is usually staphylococcal in origin but may start as molluscum contagiosum. Alternatives to look out for include infestations with scabies or lice. Herpes simplex infection may also occur, and where severe and widespread, referral to secondary care is necessary for prompt antiviral therapy.

As such, the first drugs on any prescription usually deal with the cause of the flare, antibiotics such as flucloxacillin or erythromycin to deal with an infection, and perhaps something to suppress the itch, particularly if sleep is disturbed (e.g. sedative antihistamines such as chlorphenamine, alimemazine or hydroxyzine).

Atopic eczema is a dry skin condition, and therefore the central element of all management algorithms is the copious use of emollients (despite the lack of evidence from good quality randomised controlled trials). These act by sealing the leaky skin surface to prevent the penetration of irritants and allergens, and to keep the skin hydrated which, in itself, may reduce the associated itching. Emollient therapy is perhaps best delivered by oil in the daily bath, a soap substitute for washing, and then stroking on the preferred emollient cream or ointment whilst the skin is damp, without vigorous rubbing, and allowing it to soak in. The emollient should be reapplied as often as the skin feels dry – perhaps several times a day.

Emollients, however, do not suppress inflammation. In that case, what should we use to treat inflammatory flares? Here we come to the essence of this discussion. Do we use topical corticosteroids or one of the new non-steroidal topical immunomodulators (alternatively called calcineurin inhibitors)?

Topical corticosteroids

Corticosteroid therapy has been the mainstay of treatment in atopic eczema for more than 40 years and if used properly is relatively safe and effective. Thus, for mild atopic eczema on a thick skin area, a weak corticosteroid such as 1% hydrocortisone is a safe and effective treatment, even in infants. Often, however, it is not sufficient and a stronger grade 2 or even grade 3 agent (moderately potent and potent, respectively) has to be used for a few days – less than 7 days is the current recommendation. For the face, which is far more susceptible to the adverse effects of corticosteroids (e.g. skin thinning, telangiectasia), particularly in children, potent steroids are a worry not only for the prescribing doctor, but also for patients/carers and other health workers such as health visitors and pharmacists who have had the exaggerated fears of steroids communicated to them. This irrational fear of steroids has been coined 'steroid phobia'. Working in a district general dermatological department, I am fully aware that we spend much more time encouraging patients to adequately use steroids than we ever have to curb their overuse. The skin flexures are another area of concern. A useful rule of thumb here is that the potency of the steroid used will be as effective as a grade higher because of increased absorption from these areas.

Calcineurin inhibitors

Calcineurin inhibitors are possible alternatives to prolonged exposure to topical corticosteroids, and have proven efficacy when treating problem areas (i.e. the face, the neck and the flexures) and for steroid phobics. They are also useful for patients with severe and treatment-resistant disease who would otherwise need systemic therapy. They appear to have no skin-thinning potential and do not affect the blood vessels. As is the case with all new products, there is a natural reluctance to use them more extensively until we gain more experience. However, as the number of indications for these agents will increase in the future, both with regard to age limits and the types of eczema, further experience will be gained and more extensive use is likely to develop. In addition, we should not under estimate the value that our patients place on these newer products. Given the widespread steroid phobia which still persists to this day, patients may be more confident with therapy with these newer agents and as a consequence, may be less likely to become non-compliant and cease treatment before clearance is achieved.

If we think back to our patient whose acute presentation has been dealt with, do we now send them away and wait for their next exacerbation before treating them again? Historically, the answer has been a resounding yes! However, there are a number of good studies, which demonstrate that the calcineurin inhibitors, when applied at the first signs of a flare when the skin becomes sore, itchy or red, can abort the flare. With repeated application the number of flares is also significantly reduced. Such an approach would avoid any unnecessary delay in treatment and limit the number of additional consultations and referrals into secondary care, both of which are time consuming and costly. More importantly, this technique has the potential to transform the lives of our patients. Despite this, it should be emphasised that it does take time and effort initially to educate the patient and/or parent, which is obviously much more difficult in everyday practice than it is in a clinical trial setting. This is where trained nurses can be particularly helpful, especially because support and reinforcement is so necessary. The concept of using an emollient to keep the skin healthy and a tube of prevention cream (i.e. a topical calcineurin inhibitor) to use when necessary and only resorting to a potent corticosteroid if it becomes too severe, will take time to be fully understood and accepted in practice.

Pimecrolimus is indicated for mild-to-moderate disease, whereas tacrolimus appears to be more potent and more effective in moderate-to-severe eczema. In addition, tacrolimus has been used as an alternative to a potent steroid in secondary or intermediate care. The recent National Institute for Clinical Excellence (NICE) guidelines in the UK recommend that both agents are used only by physicians (including GPs) with a special interest and experience in dermatology. The availability of two different strengths of tacrolimus ointment means that we can tailor treatment to the clinical condition of the patient, in much the same way that we use topical corticosteroids. This technique means that over time we can reduce ointment usage and thus reduce treatment costs without compromising clinical efficacy.

> Calcineurin inhibitors, when applied at the first signs of a flare when the skin becomes sore, itchy or red, can abort the flare. With repeated application the number of flares is also significantly reduced.

Constraints

The apparent cost of calcineurin inhibitors is likely to result in their widespread uptake being relatively slow in UK primary care. The fact that the gram-for-gram cost ratio of calcineurin inhibitors to corticosteroids is in the order of 18:1 may explain why there is a reluctance to permit all GPs to prescribe these newer agents, particularly when other prescribing costs are escalating rapidly. However, the morbidity saved and the effectiveness that has been demonstrated for these agents in the majority of patients, will make their sensible use, in the way I have described, a cost-effective option. Moreover, when we consider patients with more severe presentations of the disease and the greater clinical and psychological benefits that they achieve, it is likely that treatment with calcineurin inhibitors will be even more economically attractive. In the longer-term, I am sure that this situation will become analogous to the statin story, in which an initially 'dose-expensive' class of drugs has eventually become accepted as cost-effective and positively encouraged in primary care. Lost school/work time and family tensions are hard to quantify financially and, whilst they do not impinge on our prescribing budgets, they do make a big difference to the quality of life of our patients. Moreover, if primary care clinicians are given the opportunity to prescribe these drugs, then we will have a real chance of reducing referrals on to secondary care and thus the prospect of generating cost savings, as well as ensuring patients are being treated in the most appropriate clinical setting. Those of us who look after sufferers of atopic eczema in primary care fully understand the need for effective and acceptable treatment.

> If primary care clinicians are given the opportunity to prescribe these drugs, then we will have a real chance of reducing referrals on to secondary care and thus the prospect of generating cost savings.

Clinical audit

The collection of data regarding the number of repeat prescriptions of topical corticosteroids can be a useful, if horrifying, undertaking. Currently, clinical audit has particular relevance regarding the overuse of antibiotic/steroid combination topicals, which appear to be producing increased resistance figures. A useful assessment of patient education is the simple ratio between emollient and corticosteroid quantities with the ideal ratio being 10:1 or greater. A study questionnaire, distributed to all members of the primary healthcare team regarding attitudes to atopic eczema, or indeed skin disease in general, and its treatment in particular, may lead to a productive discussion so that the patient receives the same message from all, and not conflicting advice which can confuse.

Support

Support is vital for patients and their families with this chronic relapsing incurable condition, which has the ability to ruin lives and families, but can nearly always be controlled. In the UK, the National Eczema Society helpline (0870 241 3604) is a useful source of support.

In terms of professional support, here in the UK GPs can access information from the Primary Care Dermatology Society (PCDS), whilst the joint PCDS and British Association of Dermatologists atopic eczema guidelines (due for revision shortly) are available at *www.pcds.org.uk*. The PCDS also offers a range of educational meetings for its members at venues around the country and provides a quarterly bulletin. There are Diploma courses for GPs in Cardiff and London, and

> Support is vital for patients and their families with this chronic relapsing incurable condition.

examination for a diploma in Glasgow (more details are available at the PCDS website). In addition, primary care nurses have just been provided with a specific course, initially based at Southampton University but with national coverage expected to be rolled out in the future. Details about this course can be accessed from the British Dermatological Nursing Group website *(www.bdng.org.uk).*

Conclusion

The addition of calcineurin inhibitors has made a significant contribution to our armament of treatment options for the management of atopic eczema and promises much if only we are allowed and encouraged to use them. Then we can change the traditional pattern of fire-fighting acute exacerbations into a scenario where patients avoid such distress by effective prevention.

Not only are there new and effective ways of treating atopic eczema at early signs and symptoms of a flare, but treating atopic eczema earlier in life and more effectively holds the intriguing possibility that fewer children would go on to develop asthma and allergic rhinitis, a frequently observed phenomenon called the atopic march. In addition, treating more severely affected patients during childhood may prevent the likelihood of the condition persisting into adulthood. The pathophysiological link between atopic dermatitis and other atopic diseases is currently being investigated with potentially exciting implications for the future management of atopic disease. If this hypothesis is confirmed in subsequent studies, it will give even greater impetus to the compelling arguments in favour of the proactive management of atopic dermatitis.

The addition of calcineurin inhibitors has made a significant contribution to our armament of treatment options for the management of atopic eczema.

Key points

- Atopic eczema is a highly prevalent condition, particularly in childhood, with the average UK GP seeing about one patient with the condition during each surgery.

- Organised care, for example by establishing a repeat prescription service, may go a long way towards improving patient management.

- Whilst accurate diagnosis of atopic eczema is relatively straightforward, there are a number of other diagnoses that should be considered, which may impact on patient management. In addition, more severe presentations of the disease also make the disease more challenging to treat.

- Atopic eczema has a major impact on the quality of life of the patient and their families. More extensive disease impacts to a greater extent on psychosocial factors and may lead to withdrawal from leisure activities and social isolation.

- Clinical assessment and management plans are a recommended tool to record patients' progress and also provide a means of education and support.

- Lifestyle modification can control exacerbations of the condition, but pharmacological intervention is often required to maintain control of the disease. This usually takes the form of emollients and topical corticosteroids, although the availability of novel calcineurin inhibitors offer the promise of good efficacy and superior tolerability.

PATIENT NOTES
Dr Tim Mitchell

Atopic eczema – an important but neglected condition

Atopic eczema is a common and often chronic disease that has been neglected by those charged with setting new standards and targets as measures of successful treatment in the health service. Quality of life studies have shown that eczema can have as profound an effect on an individual as conditions such as diabetes and heart failure. So why do so many patients with eczema feel so dissatisfied by the level of care they are given?

Education, education, education

Skin problems are still seen as 'unimportant' or even 'cosmetic' by many people, including healthcare professionals. This arises partly from the lack of training that clinicians are given at undergraduate and postgraduate level in all areas of skin disease and basic skin care. Perhaps because of this, we are very fortunate in the UK to have excellent patient support groups that have combined together as the Skin Care Campaign to act as a powerful lobbying force. This will lead to a greater emphasis on the needs of patients with atopic eczema.

As Dr Kownacki has shown, improving the care of skin disorders such as atopic eczema should be quite straightforward as the main investment needed is in education for healthcare professionals, rather than in expensive equipment or technology. It is very important that these improvements in practice are driven by the needs of patients so that they will produce real improvements in quality of life. It is worth looking in more detail at what patients need and this has been made easier by a study which reported last year.

The International Study of Life with Atopic Eczema

This study, known as ISOLATE, revolved around interviews carried out with 2000 patients and carers in eight different countries: France, UK, Germany, Poland, the Netherlands, Spain, Mexico and the USA. Sixty per cent of those interviewed had atopic eczema with the other 40% being carers of children with the disease. The main findings of the study are summarised below.

- 75% of patients/carers said that being able to control their eczema effectively would be the single most important improvement to their quality of life.

It is very important that improvements in practice are driven by the needs of patients so that they will produce real improvements in quality of life.

- 55% admitted to worrying about the next flare-up (with 36% sometimes worrying and 19% always worrying).
- Patients with moderate eczema spent an average of 97 days each year in flare-up, whilst for those with severe eczema this figure increased to 146 days.
- 66% of patients/carers used topical steroids only as a last resort. 58% restricted their use to certain body areas due to concerns about treatment-related side-effects, and for the same reason, 39% used them less frequently than their doctor recommended.
- 67% of patients/carers said that their preferred treatment option was to apply a non-steroid treatment as early as possible to prevent a flare-up.

These findings seem to provide good evidence that patients do want alternatives to steroids and something they can use to prevent a flare-up progressing. Other findings of the study confirmed the impact that atopic eczema can have on all aspects of life:

- 33% said that eczema had impacted on their work/school, home and social life
- 14% said that their career progression had been affected by eczema, whether through limitation of choice of career or poor performance at interview
- 36% found that flare-ups affected their self-confidence
- 51% felt unhappy or depressed during flare-ups
- 21% admitted to difficulties in forming relationships
- 41% of those in established relationships said they felt awkward about partners seeing or touching their bodies
- 30% of patients and carers said that eczema had an impact on the lives of other members of the household
- only 26% said that their doctor had discussed the emotional impact of eczema with them.

The findings of the ISOLATE study should make people sit up and think about how the situation can be improved. Nationally, governments need to recognise the increasing prevalence of eczema and facilitate further research into its causes and in new approaches to treatment. At basic primary care level, healthcare staff need to acknowledge that patients need much more than just a prescription for various creams.

How can care be improved?

Many years ago it was recognised that primary care health services could provide a very good service for patients with chronic diseases such as asthma and diabetes. These proved to be so successful that they became incorporated into National Service Frameworks (NSFs) and quality standards, and their principles were extended to other areas such as heart disease. There is no

Patients do want alternatives to steroids and something they can use to prevent a flare-up progressing.

reason why this should not extend to atopic eczema and other common chronic problems such as psoriasis and acne. Most of the ongoing care is given by nurses who build up an excellent rapport with patients. I have often heard nurses complain of their frustration when dealing with a patient with asthma who also has eczema but are unable to answer their questions about the skin problem. This is not for a lack of willingness to help, and it comes back to the problem of education.

What constitutes best practice?

The following elements should form the basis of a good service for patients with atopic eczema.

- A register of all patients in the practice who suffer from it, allowing for organisation of regular reviews and the delivery of good information about new treatment options.
- A regular review session when patients can simply talk about their eczema; protected time when they can feel confident that they are not 'wasting anyone's time'.
- An acknowledgment of the impact of the disease and the need for a sense of control; this involves lots of education about the condition and the various treatments available so that patients can make well-informed choices about its management.
- Ready access to a nurse or doctor at times of flare-up or other significant events.
- Good links with secondary care to ensure current 'best practice' is followed and access to a consultant is available when it is needed, rather than through a waiting list system; this should include access to specialists in counselling and psychological care and not just dermatologists.
- Continuing professional development for all healthcare staff.

No huge investment is necessary for all this to happen, just the recognition that, as atopic eczema can account for around 5% of the total workload in primary care, those providing the care should be as well trained in this field as they are in diabetes, asthma, blood pressure and heart problems. It is only then that best use will be made of existing treatments and new treatments will be given the best chance of showing that they are very worthwhile additions to the current 'armamentarium' used in the fight against atopic eczema.

Those providing the care of eczema should be as well trained in this field as they are in diabetes, asthma, blood pressure and heart problems.

Glossary

Absorption – The movement and uptake of a drug into cells or across tissues (such as the skin, intestine and kidney).

Acanthosis – Abnormal thickening and darkening of areas of the skin.

Acaricidal sprays – Chemical sprays that are used to kill mites and ticks (small, blood-sucking parasites).

Acne – A skin disorder characterised by inflammation of the hair follicles and sebaceous (oil) glands, leading to the formation of blackheads, pimples and pustules. Acne is one of the most common skin disorders and is particularly common amongst children and young adults.

Acute – A relatively short course of drug treatment lasting days or weeks rather than months. Can also refer to the duration of a disease or condition.

Acute lesions – An area of sore or infected skin that develops suddenly and lasts for a short period of time.

Adverse event – An unwanted reaction to a medical treatment.

Aeroallergens – Allergens that are carried in the air, such as dust and pollen.

Aetiology – The specific causes or origins of a disease, usually a result of both genetic and environmental factors.

Agranulocytosis – A disorder of the blood characterised by a dramatic reduction in the number of granulocytes (a type of white blood cell). As a result, the patient has little resistance to infection. The disorder is commonly caused by radiation therapy and the use of certain drugs (e.g. sulphonamides). Treatment involves the use of antibiotics and steroids, and blood transfusions to supply white blood cells.

Allergens – Substances that cause an allergic reaction in the body. Common allergens include dust, animal hair and fur (dander), pollen and peanuts.

Allergic rhinitis – The medical term for hay fever. Inflammation of the nasal passages in response to an allergic stimulus (e.g. pollen, mould, dust mites, animal dander). Symptoms often include sneezing and a blocked, runny or itchy nose. Allergic rhinitis can be intermittent, occurring at specific times of the year (i.e. during the pollen seasons in the spring and autumn), or persistent, with sufferers experiencing symptoms all year round.

Ammonium lactate – A skin moisturiser that is available as a cream or lotion and is used to treat dry, scaly skin conditions.

Anabolic – Pertaining to anabolism, the build-up or synthesis of molecules within the body. The build up of proteins in the body leading to the development of muscle is an example of anabolism.

Antecubital – Pertaining to the region of the arm located in front of the elbow.

Antibody – Proteins present in the blood that target and destroy particular antigens.

Antigen – Any foreign substance within the body that stimulates an immune response.

Antihistamines – See H_1-receptor antagonists. Drugs that are used in the treatment of allergic reactions, including allergic rhinitis (hay fever), insect bites and the emergency treatment of anaphylaxis (a life-threatening allergic reaction in which breathing is severely compromised). Antihistamines work by blocking the action of histamine, a substance that is released during an allergic reaction and causes swelling and itching. The newer antihistamines (e.g. desloratadine, fexofenadine, levocetirizine, loratadine, terfenadine) do not cause as much drowsiness as the older drugs.

Antimicrobial – An agent that kills or impedes the growth and reproduction of microbes, including bacteria, viruses and fungi.

Antipruritic – An agent that relieves itching.

Apoptosis – The death of cells through a programmed sequence of events. This is a normal and essential process that occurs throughout the body and is a means by which the body gets rid of damaged or unwanted cells.

Ascomycin – A drug that is used topically (applied to the surface of the skin) for the treatment of atopic dermatitis (eczema).

Asteatotic eczema – A type of eczema that mainly affects older people. Commonly known as winter eczema or winter itch, asteatotic eczema is aggravated by cold, dry air, central heating and winter clothing. It commonly affects the limbs (particularly the shins) and is characterised by peeling and cracking of the skin.

Atopic – Suffering from atopy.

Atopic dermatitis – Also known as atopic eczema. An allergic skin disorder that frequently occurs in babies and young children who are atopic. The condition is characterised by inflamed, itchy, flaky skin, and tends to affect the face, elbows, knees and arms. Usually disappears around the age of 3 or 4 years but can persist into adolescence and adulthood.

Atopic Dermatitis Severity Index (ADSI) – A scale for measuring the severity of atopic dermatitis. A four-point scale is used to grade the severity of skin erythema (reddening), pruritus (itching), exudation (leaking fluid), excoriation (scratches or breaks in the skin) and lichenification (thickening). The sum of these ratings provides the total score. The ADSI is used in clinical trials to evaluate the effectiveness of potential eczema treatments.

Atopy – The tendency to suffer from allergies, such as asthma, eczema and hay fever. Atopy is commonly inherited.

Atopy patch test – A skin test used to identify allergies. A purified preparation of the potential allergen (e.g. pet hair, house-dust mite or grass pollen) is secured to the skin on the upper back. The allergen is left in contact with the skin for up to 72 hours. The appearance and the number and distribution pattern of any resulting skin lesions are then examined.

Atrophogenic – Causing atrophy, the wasting away of a tissue or organ.

Avidity – The strength of binding between two molecules or two cells. Often used to describe the strength with which an antibody binds to a particular antigen.

B cells – A type of white blood cell that produces antibodies (proteins that help to defend the body against foreign substances). Also known as B lymphocytes.

Baseline – The starting point to which all subsequent measurements are compared. Used as a means of assessing improvement or deterioration over the course of a clinical trial.

Betamethasone valerate – A corticosteroid with anti-inflammatory properties that is applied topically (to the surface of the skin) for the treatment of inflammatory skin conditions, such as eczema and psoriasis.

Bioavailability – The amount of a drug that enters the bloodstream and hence reaches the tissues and organs of the body. Usually expressed as a percentage of the dose given.

Binding – The force with which two molecules are attracted to each other and held together.

Blood stem cells – Immature, unspecialised cells located in the bone marrow, from which all other types of blood cell are formed.

Calcineurin – A phosphatase enzyme that plays an important role in the body's immune response by controlling the production of inflammatory cytokines by activated T lymphocytes. The calcineurin inhibitors (e.g. pimecrolimus and tacrolimus) represent a non-steroidal alternative for the treatment of eczema.

Carcinogen – A substance capable of causing cancer.

Cardiomyopathy – A general term for any disease of the heart muscle that results in the heart being unable to pump blood around the body properly.

Cataract – Partial or complete clouding of the lens of the eye, leading to blurred vision and in extreme cases, blindness.

Cell nucleus – The part of a cell that contains the genetic material. Plural; nuclei.

Ceramides – Naturally occurring fats that help to protect the skin from water loss by forming a protective barrier. Ceramides can also be produced synthetically and are added to some skin care products.

Chlorphenamine – An antihistamine that is used to treat allergic conditions, such as hay fever and urticaria (itchy, raised lumps on the skin due to an allergic reaction; also known as hives). Chlorphenamine is a 'sedating antihistamine' and as such, can cause drowsiness.

Cholesterol – A fat-like substance found in blood and all body cells and used in the manufacture of cell membranes and hormones. A high level of cholesterol in the blood is a major risk factor for heart disease.

Chronic – A prolonged course of drug treatment lasting months rather than weeks. Can also refer to the duration of a disease or condition.

Ciclosporin – Also known as cyclosporin. A drug that suppresses the body's immune system by inhibiting calcineurin. Ciclosporin is used in patients who have undergone an organ transplant to prevent the body from rejecting the new organ. It also slows skin cell growth and can also be used to treat inflammatory skin conditions, such as eczema and psoriasis when they are very severe.

Coadministration – The simultaneous administration of more than one type of medication.

Coal tar – A thick, black, opaque liquid that is a by-product of the conversion of coal into coke. Used in the production of many substances, including creams, lotions and bath products for the treatment of eczema and psoriasis.

Collagen synthesis – The production of collagen, the main protein in skin, tendons, ligaments, bone, cartilage and connective tissue. Collagen provides strength and resilience to these tissues.

Comorbid – A co-existing medical condition.

Conjunctiva – The thin, clear membrane that covers the eyeball and the undersurface of the eyelids.

Connective tissue – The tissues in the body that provide support, such as bone, tendons, ligaments and fat tissue.

Contact eczema – An allergic reaction in the skin caused by contact of the skin with a particular chemical or other irritant (e.g. jewellery, drug, cleaning product, washing powder). Characterised by dry, itchy and flaky skin that may become cracked, red and inflamed.

Contraindication – Specific circumstances under which a drug should not be prescribed, for example, certain drugs should not be given simultaneously.

Corticosteroids – Hormones produced by the adrenal glands. These compounds can be used to treat a variety of inflammatory conditions, including asthma, rheumatoid arthritis, eczema and hay fever. They can also be used to prevent the rejection of a transplanted organ.

Cosmetic acne – Acne caused by exposure to cosmetics that contain certain ingredients.

Creatinine – A protein produced from the breakdown of creatine by the muscle. Creatinine is released from the muscle into the blood, and is cleared from the blood via the kidneys. Levels of creatinine in the blood and the rate at which it is cleared from the blood are used as indicators of kidney function.

Crotamiton – A drug that is used to treat pruritis (itching of the skin). When applied to the skin, crotamiton evaporates rapidly, producing a cooling effect. Often used to treat the itching caused by eczema, psoriasis and scabies.

Cushing's syndrome – A hormonal disorder caused by abnormally high levels of corticosteroid hormones in the blood, owing to overactivity of the adrenal glands or pituitary gland, or by the prolonged use of corticosteroid drugs. Patients with Cushing's syndrome have a characteristic round, red face, an obese trunk, a humped upper back and wasted limbs.

Cutaneous – Pertaining to the skin.

Cytochrome P450 (CYP) enzymes – A family of enzymes found in the liver that play an important role in the metabolism and detoxification of various compounds, including many drugs.

Cytokine gene – A gene (segment of DNA on a chromosome) that controls the production of cytokines.

Cytokine mediators – See Cytokines.

Cytokines – Small protein messengers secreted by immune cells (e.g. macrophages, monocytes, lymphocytes and neutrophils) in response to a stimulus, that affect the behaviour of other nearby cells. Examples of cytokines include histamine, prostaglandins, tumour necrosis factor (TNF) and the interleukins (IL).

Cytosol – The thick fluid contained within a cell in which all the different parts of the cell are suspended. Contains enzymes for metabolic reactions together with sugars, salts, amino acids, nucleotides and everything else needed for the cell to function.

Cytosolic nuclear factors – Proteins found in the cytosol of a cell that control the transport of molecules into and out of the cell nucleus.

Cytosolic proteins – Proteins that are present in the cytosol of a cell.

Cytotoxic T cells – A type of T lymphocyte; white blood cells found in blood and the lymphatic system. Play a major role in the body's immune response, by binding to and destroying foreign cells, such as bacteria, viruses and tumour cells. There are a number of different types of T lymphocyte, including cytotoxic T cells, helper T cells, suppressor T cells and regulatory T cells.

Degranulation – The release of the contents of secretory granules from a cell. For example, during an allergic reaction, mast cells (cells that play a role in allergic reactions, wound healing and the sensation of itching) release histamine, cytokines, enzymes and prostaglandins.

Dephosphorylating – Causing the removal of phosphate groups (PO_4) from a molecule.

Depigmentation – The removal or loss of skin pigments (e.g. melanin) leading to pale spots on the skin.

Dermal – Pertaining to the dermis of the skin.

Dermal mast cells – Cells found in the dermis that play a role in allergic reactions, wound healing and itching. Activated when they come into contact with allergens, mast cells release various substances, including histamine, cytokines, enzymes and prostaglandins.

Dermatitis – Inflammation of the skin. Symptoms include redness, itching and sometimes scaling.

Dermatoses – Diseases of the skin.

Dermis – The layer of skin below the surface (epidermis) of the skin.

Discoid eczema – A chronic form of dermatitis that is characterised by coin- or disc-shaped areas of inflammation. Tends to affect the arms and legs of middle-aged adults, and is usually worse in the winter than in the summer.

Dizygotic – Arising from two separately fertilised eggs.

DNA – Deoxyribonucleic acid. The molecule found in the nucleus of cells that stores the genetic information for each individual. Determines the structure, function and behaviour of the cell. Comprised of two strands of nucleotides coiled together as a double helix. In 1962, James Watson, Francis Crick and Maurice Wilkins received the Nobel Prize for their model of the structure of DNA.

Dose-finding study – A clinical trial designed to determine the optimum dose of a drug (the dose that is clinically effective without causing excessive side-effects).

Dose-ranging study – A clinical trial designed to determine the range of doses between which a drug is clinically effective.

Double-blind – A clinical trial in which neither the doctor nor the patient are aware of the treatment allocation.

Down regulate – Slow down or suppress.

Drop-out rates – The number of patients who fail to complete a clinical trial. Possible reasons can include unacceptable side-effects and moving away from the area where the trial is being conducted.

Drug interactions – In which the action of one drug interferes with that of another, with potentially hazardous consequences. Interactions are particularly common when the patient is taking more than one form of medication for the treatment of multiple disease states or conditions.

Eczema molluscatum – Eczema infected with the pox virus *Molluscum contagiosum.* Leads to the development of brick-shaped bumps on the infected skin.

Eczematous – Having the characteristics of eczema.

Efficacy – The effectiveness of a drug against the disease or condition it was designed to treat.

Electrolyte – A substance that dissolves in water to form ions which are able to conduct electricity. Examples of electrolytes are sodium and potassium salts. These dissolve in water to produce sodium and potassium ions, respectively.

Emollients – Substances composed of fat or oil that soften and soothe the skin.

Endogenous – Manufactured within the body.

Endothelial cells – Multifunctional cells that line blood vessels. Functions include: acting as a barrier between blood and other body tissues; attracting white blood cells to the site of an infection; regulating blood flow; regulating blood clotting; controlling the contraction and relaxation of veins. The endothelial cells are collectively called the endothelium of the blood vessel.

Endpoint – A recognised stage in the disease process, used to compare the outcome in the different treatment arms of clinical trials. Endpoints can mark improvement or deterioration of the patient and signify the end of the trial.

Enterotoxins – Substances that are toxic to the gastrointestinal tract. May cause nausea, vomiting, cramps and diarrhoea.

Enzyme – A protein produced by cells in the body that catalyses a specific biochemical reaction but is itself not used up in the process.

Eosinophils – White blood cells that destroy foreign organisms in the body and play a major role in allergic reactions. Eosinophils also secrete chemical mediators (e.g. eosinophilic cationic protein [ECP]) that can cause bronchoconstriction in asthma. Characterised by the presence of coarse granules in their cytoplasm and found in large numbers in the mucosa (the lining of the body passages and cavities that connect with the exterior).

Epidemiology – The incidence or distribution of a disease within a population.

Epidermal – Pertaining to the epidermis.

Epidermal dendritic cells – A type of cell present in the skin. Use thread-like tentacles to trap antigens, and thus initiate an immune response.

Epidermal lipid synthesis – The production of lipids (fats) in the epidermal skin cells which help to cement skin cells together.

Epidermis – The outermost layer of skin.

Erythema – Reddening of the skin.

Erythematous – Characterised by redness of the skin.

Essential fatty acids – The building blocks of fats, fatty acids consist of a long chain of carbon and hydrogen atoms attached to a carboxylic acid group (COOH). Essential fatty acids cannot be produced in the body, and must therefore be obtained from the diet. Examples include linoleic and linolenic acid.

Exacerbation – A period during which the symptoms of a disease recur or become worse. Commonly used to describe an asthma attack.

Excipients – Inactive ingredients that are added to drugs to give stability or bulk so that the drug can be manufactured as required (e.g. as a tablet).

Excoriations – Scratches or breaks in the skin.

Excretion – The elimination of a drug or substance from the body as a waste product, for example, in the urine or faeces.

Exudation – The leakage/discharge of fluid from blood vessels in response to inflammation.

Exudative – Pertaining to the process of exudation.

FcεRI – A receptor to which immunoglobulin E (IgE) antibodies bind strongly. Present on the surface of certain immune cells (mast cells, basophils, eosinophils and monocytes) and Langherans (dendritic) cells in the skin. Plays a central role in allergic reactions.

Fibroblasts – Cells involved in the production of connective tissue (the tissues in the body that provide support, such as bone, tendons, ligaments and fat tissue). Fibroblasts are also themselves capable of developing into connective tissue cells (e.g. bone, fat and smooth muscle cells), and can migrate to the site of an injury to repair the damaged connective tissue.

Flexural – Pertaining to a flexure.

Flexures – Folds or bends.

Follicular orifices – The sac-like openings of the hair follicles on the surface of the skin.

Folliculitis – Inflammation of hair follicles due to infection or irritation.

Free radicals – Atoms or molecules that contain an unpaired electron and are highly reactive at cellular structures, because they take electrons from other molecules to become more stable. This process, known as oxidation, is toxic to many cells and can result in cellular damage. Free radicals are the by-products of both normal and pathological processes within the body.

Gastrointestinal – Pertaining to the stomach and intestines.

Genetic predisposition – An individuals' susceptibility to develop a disease or condition as a result of their genetic or chromosomal make-up.

Glaucoma simplex – A disease in which the pressure inside the eye is raised. This causes damage to the optic nerve, leading to loss of vision and, if left untreated, blindness. Glaucoma simplex is the most common type of glaucoma and is also known as open-angle or chronic glaucoma.

Glucocorticoid – A type of corticosteroid, glucocorticoids are produced by the adrenal glands and play a key role in energy metabolism. Possess anti-inflammatory and immunosuppressive properties.

Glucocorticoid response elements – Sequences of DNA in the nucleus of a cell to which the complex of a glucocorticoid and its receptor binds. This binding then activates transcription (the copying of a sequence of DNA into messenger RNA, which serves as a blueprint for the synthesis of a particular protein).

Graft-versus-host disease – A condition that can occur after a person has undergone a bone marrow transplant. The immune cells in the donor bone marrow produce antibodies against the transplant patient's tissues, and these attack the patient's organs. Severe cases of the disease can be fatal. Immune suppressants (e.g. high doses of corticosteroids) are used to suppress or prevent graft-*versus*-host disease.

Graft-versus-host reaction – See Graft-*versus*-host disease.

Granulocyte-macrophage colony-stimulating factor (GM-CSF) – A naturally occurring glycoprotein (a protein with carbohydrate molecules attached to it) that is produced at sites of inflammation. Stimulates bone marrow cells to produce certain types of white blood cell (granulocytes and macrophages). Also used as a drug to stimulate the production of white blood cells in patients whose immune system is not working properly (e.g. patients receiving chemotherapy or bone marrow transplant patients).

H$_1$-receptor antagonists – See Antihistamines.

H$_1$-receptors – Proteins on the surface of cells that mediate the biological effects of histamine. Activation of H$_1$ receptors leads to the symptoms associated with allergic reactions, such as sneezing and itching.

Heavy metals – A group of elements that can produce toxic effects at low concentrations. Examples include mercury, lead, zinc, iron and copper.

Hepatic – Pertaining to the liver.

Hepato- – Pertaining to the liver.

Herpes simplex – A virus. Infection with herpes simplex can lead to the formation of blister-like sores on the face, lips, mouth or genitals.

Hexosaminidase – An enzyme that breaks down fatty substances in the brain and nerves. A deficiency of this enzyme causes Tay-Sachs disease, a fatal neurological disorder, for which there is no cure.

High affinity – Describes a substance that binds (attaches) strongly to its target, such as a receptor.

High-affinity receptor – A protein on the surface of cells that binds (attaches) strongly to a particular chemical or drug.

Histamine – An inflammatory substance that is released from mast cells during an allergic reaction. Histamine is one of the substances responsible for the swelling and redness associated with inflammation. Other effects include narrowing of the airways, itching and the stimulation of acid production in the stomach. The effects of histamine can be counteracted with antihistamine drugs (e.g. levocetirizine, desloratadine and loratadine).

Histopathological – Pertaining to histopathology, the microscopic study of diseased cells and tissues.

Homeopathy – A system of natural medicine in which very small doses of a substance that stimulates symptoms of a particular disease are used to heal the same symptoms in a sick person by stimulating the body's own defence and healing processes.

Humectants – Substances that help to moisturise the skin by drawing moisture from the air.

Hydrate – To add moisture (water).

Hyperaesthesia – Abnormally increased sensory perception.

Hyperkeratosis – Thickening and hardening of the outer layer of the skin.

Hypertension – Excessively high blood pressure.

Hypertrichosis – Excessive body hair.

Hypomagnesaemic – Having a magnesium deficiency.

Hypopigmentation – A lack of skin colour, resulting in skin that is lighter than normal. Caused by a deficiency of melanin in the skin.

Hypothalamic–pituitary–adrenal (HPA) axis – The interaction between the hypothalamus, the pituitary gland and the adrenal glands. The hypothalamus lies just above the pituitary gland in the brain. It releases corticotropin-releasing hormone (CRH), which stimulates the pituitary gland to release adrenocorticotrophic hormone (ACTH). This, in turn, stimulates the adrenal glands to secrete corticosteroid hormones, which play an important role in the regulation of fat, protein and carbohydrate metabolism, and in suppressing inflammatory reactions in the body.

Ichthammol paste – A paste containing ichthammol that is used to relieve the itching associated with eczema. Ichthammol is an oily by-product from the conversion of coal into coke.

IgE antibodies – Protein–sugar complexes known as immunoglobulins that are produced by the body in response to the presence of an antigen (a foreign substance such as a virus or bacterium) and combine with the foreign substance to make it harmless. Antibodies are produced by certain white blood cells (B cells), and circulate in the blood and tissue fluids. Antibodies are grouped into five classes: IgA, IgD, IgE, IgG and IgM. IgE antibodies are the major antibodies involved in allergic reactions.

IL-10 receptors – Proteins on the surface of a cell that act as a binding site for the cytokine, interleukin (IL)-10, and mediate its biological effects.

IL-4 – One of a family of 12 cytokines. IL-4 plays a key role in allergic reactions.

Immunoglobulin (Ig) antibodies – Protein–sugar complexes that are produced by the body in response to the presence of an antigen (a foreign substance, such as a virus or bacterium). Antibodies are produced by certain white blood cells (B cells) and circulate in the blood and tissue fluids. The antibodies combine with the foreign substance to make it harmless. Antibodies are grouped into five classes: IgG, IgA, IgM, IgD and IgE. IgE antibodies are the main antibodies involved in allergic reactions.

Immunoglobulin E (IgE) – One of the five classes of antibody produced in the body. Immunoglobulin E antibodies play a key role in the body's allergic response.

Immunohistochemical – Pertaining to immunohistochemistry, the microscopic examination of cells and tissues that have been stained using specific antibodies.

Immunomodulators – Substances that alter the activity of the body's immune system.

Immunomodulatory agents – See Immunomodulators.

Immunophilins – Receptors targeted by drugs that suppress the body's immune system, such as ciclosporin.

Immunosuppressant – Substances that suppress the body's immune response (e.g. ciclosporin). Used in patients who have undergone an organ transplant in order to prevent the body from rejecting the new organ.

Immunosurveillance – The mechanisms by which the immune system is able to recognise and destroy malignant cells.

Impetigo – A bacterial skin infection characterised by small, pus-filled blisters usually located on the face, about the nose and mouth. Most common in children.

Induration – Abnormal hardening of a soft tissue.

Inflammatory dendritic epidermal cells (IDEC) – A cell present in skin that is affected by atopic eczema. The cells express the FcεR1 receptor, which has a high affinity for immunoglobulin E (IgE) antibodies. IDEC are thought to play a central role in the inflammation associated with atopic eczema.

Intercellular adhesion molecule (ICAM)-1 – A receptor present on the surface of cells of the immune system. Helps these cells to stick to the surface of other cells and thereby plays a key role in immune and inflammatory processes.

Interferon (IFN)-γ – A substance produced by white blood cells that helps the body to fight infections and tumours. In particular, it has antiviral properties.

Interleukins (IL) – A family of cytokines produced by white blood cells that play an important role in the functioning of the body's immune system. Twelve different interleukins have been identified, all with differing roles. For example, IL-4 plays a role in allergic reactions, IL-1, IL-6 and IL-11 are involved in the production of certain proteins by the liver in response to inflammation, and IL-9 stimulates mast cells to release histamine.

Intractable atopic eczema – Atopic eczema that does not respond to treatment and is difficult to control.

In vitro – 'In glass'. Used with reference to experiments performed outside the living system in a laboratory setting.

In vivo – Used with reference to experiments performed within the living cell or organism.

Irradiation – Treatment with low levels of radiation, such as X-rays, gamma rays and ultraviolet rays, for medical purposes (e.g. to reduce the presence of disease-causing agents).

Isoenzyme – One of a group of related enzymes that catalyse the same biochemical reaction but differ in their structure and biochemical properties.

Keratinocytes – The main type of cell in the outer layer of the skin. Produce the protein, keratin.

Langerhans cells – A type of dendritic cell found in the skin. Dendritic cells use thread-like tentacles to trap antigens, and thus initiate an immune response.

Lesions – Wounds or injury to the skin.

Leukocytes – The collective name for white blood cells. White blood cells are found in the blood and lymphatic system, where they help the body to fight infections and disease. There are three types of white blood cell: granulocytes, lymphocytes and monocytes.

Lichen planus – A skin disease characterised by small, shiny, flat-topped pink or purple spots on the arms or legs. Can also affect the mouth.

Lichenification – Thickening of the skin.

Linoleic acid – An essential fatty acid.

Linolenic acid – An essential fatty acid.

Lipids – Fats and fat-like substances which are insoluble in water yet dissolve freely in non-polar solvents (e.g. alcohol). All lipids contain aliphatic hydrocarbons.

Lipophilic – Having a tendency to dissolve in fat. The term literally means 'fat-loving'. Examples of lipophilic molecules include oils and fats.

Lipophilicity – The extent to which a molecule or part of a molecule is lipophilic.

Locus – The position on a chromosome where the gene for a particular trait is located.

Lymphatic system – The tissues and organs (including the bone marrow, spleen, thymus and lymph nodes) that manufacture and store the cells that fight infection.

Macrolactams – A group of non-steroidal agents that suppress the immune system and are used for the topical treatment of atopic dermatitis and other dermatoses. Pimecrolimus and tacrolimus are macrolactams.

Macrolides – A group of antibacterial drugs whose activity is due to the presence of a 'macrolide' ring in their chemical structure. Examples include erythromycin, azithromycin and clarithromycin.

Macrophages – Cells that form part of the immune system. Found mainly in the liver and lymph nodes, macrophages are responsible for clearing the blood and other tissues of foreign particles, such as bacteria and dead cells.

Macrophillin-12 (FKBP-12) – A protein found on T lymphocytes that acts as a receptor for immunosuppressive drugs (e.g. tacrolimus and pimecrolimus).

Malassezia furfur – Formerly known as *Pityrosporum ovale*. A yeast that is found naturally on the surface of the skin. The most common cause of dandruff.

Mast cell – A cell that releases histamine and other chemicals involved in inflammation. Mast cells are responsible for the immediate reddening of the skin after an allergic response.

Mechanism of action – The manner in which a drug exerts its therapeutic effects.

Messenger RNA (mRNA) – A molecule that acts as a template for the manufacture of specific proteins. Copied from the DNA in the nucleus of the cell, mRNA then travels from the nucleus into the cytoplasm, where it directs the synthesis of the protein described by that particular gene.

Meta-analysis – A set of statistical procedures designed to amalgamate the results from a number of different clinical studies. Meta-analyses provide a more accurate representation of a particular clinical situation than is provided by individual clinical studies.

Metabolism – The process by which a drug is broken down within the body.

Metabolites – The products of metabolism.

Microbial colonisation – The multiplication of microbes (microscopic organisms, such as viruses, bacteria and fungi) within a particular environment.

Microflora – Microscopic plant life, including viruses, bacteria, yeasts and fungi.

Molluscum contagiosum – A pox virus that can cause eczema molluscatum; a type of eczema characterised by brick-shaped bumps on the infected skin.

Monocyte chemoattractant protein (MCP)-1 – A protein that attracts monocytes to sites of injury and infection.

Monocytes – A type of white blood cell. Enlarge and develop into macrophages.

Monotherapy – Treatment with a single drug.

Monozygotic – Arising from one fertilised egg.

Morbidity – A diseased condition or state, or the incidence of a disease within a population.
Morphological – Pertaining to morphology.
Morphology – The physical shape, size, form and structure of animals and plants.
Mortality – The death rate of a population. The ratio of the total number of deaths to the total population.
Multicentre – A clinical trial conducted across a number of treatment centres, either abroad or in the same country.
Multifactorial – A disease or state arising from more than one causative element.
Myalgia – Pain in the muscles.
Natural killer (NK) cells – A type of white blood cell that destroys infected abnormal cells (e.g. tumour cells) in the body.
Nephrotoxicity – Being harmful to the kidneys.
Netherton's syndrome – A rare skin disease of unknown cause. Usually present at birth and often associated with failure to thrive in infancy. Characterised by flaking skin, red rashes, sparse hair growth and fragile 'bamboo' hair (hair that is not smooth like normal hair but has nodules along its length).
Neurogenic – Originating in the nerves, or stimulated by nerves.
Neuropeptides – A family of small proteins that act as neurotransmitters (e.g. substance P, tachykinins, calcitonin gene-related peptide [CGRP]). Contribute to inflammatory reactions, for example, substance P and the tachykinins produce smooth muscle contraction and mucus secretion.
Neutral pH – A pH value of 7, indicating that the solution in question contains equal concentrations of hydrogen (H^+) and hydroxide (OH^-) ions and is therefore neither acidic nor alkaline.
Occlusive – Being obstructive or impenetrable. The term is often used to describe a dressing that is applied to damaged skin in order to prevent or slow moisture evaporation.
Oedematous – Having the property of oedema; the accumulation of excessive fluid in the tissues, leading to swelling.
Open-label – A clinical trial in which all participants (i.e. the doctor and the patient) are aware of the treatment allocation.
p53 – A protein that suppresses the growth of tumour cells. Many types of cancer are thought to be due to a deficiency in this protein.
pH – A measure of the concentration of hydrogen ions (hydrogen atoms with a single positive charge due to the loss of one negatively charged electron) in a solution. The greater the concentration of hydrogen ions, the lower the pH. A pH of less than 7 indicates an acidic solution, whilst a pH greater than 7 indicates an alkaline solution.
p-value – In statistical analysis, a measure of the probability that a given result occurred by chance. If the p-value is less than or equal to 0.05 then the result is usually considered to be statistically significant, and not due to chance.
Papulation – The formation of papules, small, solid bumps on the skin.
Parallel group – A clinical trial in which patients receive only one of the treatments being tested or compared. A separate group(s) of patients will receive the alternative treatment option(s).
Pathogen – An organism or substance that causes disease.
Pathogenesis – The processes involved in the development of a particular disease.
Pathophysiology – The functional changes that accompany a particular syndrome or disease.
Peptides – Small proteins consisting of short chains of two or more amino acids (the building blocks of proteins).
Petrolatum – Another name for petroleum jelly (Vaseline®). Used to soften and soothe the skin.

Pharmacodynamics – The physiological and biological effects of a drug, including its mechanism of action – the process by which it exerts its therapeutic effects.

Pharmacokinetics – The activity of the drug within the body over a period of time.

Pharmacology – The branch of science that deals with the origin, nature, chemistry, effects and uses of drugs.

Phosphatase – An enzyme that catalyses (speeds up) the removal of phosphate groups (PO_4) from proteins.

Photoactive – Reacting to light.

Photoallergenic – Describes a substance that may interact with light to cause an allergic reaction.

Phototoxic – A substance that may increase the sensitivity of the skin to light.

Placebo – An inert substance with no specific pharmacological activity.

Placebo-controlled – A clinical trial in which a proportion of patients are given placebo in place of the active drug.

Placental membrane – The barrier that separates the blood supply of the foetus from that of the mother. Substances circulating in the maternal blood must pass through this membrane to reach the foetal blood.

Pleiomorphic lymphoma – A tumour of the lymphatic system that consists of cells that have not yet developed into any particular cell type (undifferentiated). As a result, the tumour has the potential to turn into one of a number of different types of lymphoma.

Pneumococcal – Referring to the bacterium *Streptococcus pneumoniae*. This bacterium is present in the nose and throat of some individuals, but does not cause infection unless it is able to invade other parts of the body, such as the sinuses and lungs. Responsible for a number of infections in humans, including pneumonia, meningitis and sinusitis.

Pooled analysis – The amalgamation and processing of data derived from multiple clinical trials.

Popliteal fossa – The area on the back of the leg behind the knee.

Porcine model – A model of a human disease in a pig.

Probiotics – Non-pathogenic (not disease-causing) bacteria that are added to certain foods in order to promote health and well-being. An example is the *lactobacillus* bacterium, which can be added to milk or yogurt.

Procollagen propeptide types I and III – Two small proteins that are located on the ends of procollagen types I and III (precursor molecules to collagen, a protein synthesised in the skin). Procollagen is converted into collagen by removal of the propeptides at the ends of the molecules. Measuring the levels of the two propeptides in the blood gives an indication of the extent of collagen synthesis in the skin.

Prophylaxis – Preventative treatment. Steps taken to prevent a disease before it occurs.

Propylene glycol – A chemical consisting of glycerin and water that is added to many cosmetic products to soften and moisturise the skin. Concerns have been raised about the use of this chemical in skin products because it can cause allergies and irritation.

Pruritus – Itching.

Psoralen – A chemical that increases the skin's sensitivity to sunlight. Often used to treat psoriasis and vitiligo (white patches on the skin due to the loss of pigment-producing cells).

Psoriasis – A chronic (long-lasting or recurrent) disease of the skin characterised by raised, red, itchy, inflamed areas that may be covered with white scales. Commonly affects the scalp, arms and legs.

Psychosomatic – Physical symptoms resulting from psychological (emotional) factors.

Pyoderma gangrenosum – Rapidly developing skin ulcers with a well-defined, red, overhanging border.

Radiolabelled – Tagged with a radioactive substance. Commonly used to visualise biological processes *in vivo*.

Receptors – A molecular structure, usually situated on the cell membrane, which mediates the biological response that is associated with a particular drug or substance.

Refractory facial eczematous lesions – Areas of eczema on the face that do not respond to treatment.

Renal – Pertaining to the kidneys.

Rescue therapy – Emergency therapy that is used when a patient has not responded to the usual forms of treatment.

Respiratory distress syndrome – A condition where the person is unable to breathe in sufficient oxygen due to lung damage caused by illness or injury. As a result, blood levels of oxygen become dangerously low. The condition mainly occurs in premature babies whose lungs are not yet fully developed.

RNA transcription – The first step in the process of protein synthesis in cells, whereby the DNA in the cell nucleus is transcribed (copied) into another molecule known as RNA (ribonucleic acid) through the action of enzymes (proteins that speed up biochemical reactions in the body).

Safety and tolerability – The side-effects associated with a particular drug and the likelihood that patients will tolerate a drug treatment regimen.

Salicylic acid – The active chemical ingredient in aspirin. Salicylic acid is also used in cosmetics, as an antiseptic and preservative.

Scabies – A highly contagious skin disease in humans, wild and domestic animals, that is caused by tiny mites that burrow under the skin causing it to itch and break out into a rash of small pimples.

Scalded skin syndrome – Reddening and subsequent peeling of the skin due to infection with the bacterium *Staphylococcus aureus*. Most common in children and newborn babies.

Seborrheic dermatitis – A chronic skin condition that is characterised by inflamed, itchy, red, scaly skin on the face, scalp, chest or back. The exact cause is unknown, but it may be due to infection with the yeast, *Malassezia furfur*. Tends to develop in times of stress. Mild seborrheic dermatitis of the scalp is known as dandruff.

Secretions – Chemical substances produced and released by cells, glands or organs that are needed for metabolic processes elsewhere in the body.

Sera – Plural of serum.

Serotonin – A neurotransmitter in the brain that plays an important role in the regulation of mood, sexuality and food intake.

Serum – The clear, straw-coloured, fluid component of blood that results after the clotting agents (e.g. fibrinogen and prothrombin) have been removed.

Serum immunoglobulin E (IgE) – Levels of IgE in the serum.

Sham irradiation – Identical to the normal irradiation procedure but does not actually deliver radiation to the subject; a type of placebo (inactive) treatment.

Single-blind – A clinical trial in which only the patient is unaware of the treatment allocation.

Sinusitis – Inflammation of the membrane lining the facial sinuses (hollow cavities behind the forehead and cheekbones) due to a bacterial or viral infection, or an allergic reaction. Symptoms include pain in the face, headache, a blocked or runny nose, sensitive teeth and swelling around the eyes. The condition may be treated with decongestants (drugs that reduce nasal congestion) and, in the case of a bacterial infection, antibiotics.

Skin atrophy – Shrinkage or wasting away of the skin.

Skin barrier – The barrier provided by the skin that protects the body's internal organs from the environment (e.g. injury, sunlight and invasion by infective agents).

Skin prick test – A test used to diagnose allergies. A drop of allergen is injected into the skin using a small needle. The appearance of a small, red, itchy swelling around the site of injection indicates that the person is allergic to that particular allergen.

Socioeconomic impact – Social and economic factors that characterise the influence of a disease. Incorporates the financial cost incurred by the healthcare provider, patient and/or their employer.

Spongiosis – Inflammation of the outer layer of the skin due to the abnormal accumulation of fluid between cells.

Staphylococcal – Pertaining to the *Staphylococcus* group of bacteria.

Staphylococcus aureus – A bacterium from the *Staphylococcus* group that is present in the nasal passages, throat, hair and skin of healthy individuals. Causes a variety of infections, ranging from minor skin infections (e.g. pimples and boils), to life-threatening infections, such as meningitis, pneumonia and septicaemia (blood poisoning).

Statistical significance – A measure of the probability that a given result derived from a clinical trial – be it an improvement or a decline in the health of the patient – is due to a specific effect of drug treatment, rather than a chance occurrence.

Steroid – See Corticosteroids.

Steroidal – Pertaining to steroids or their effects.

Steroid-induced rosacea – A skin condition caused by the use of steroids. Characterised by patches of red skin with pimples and broken blood vessels on the cheeks and nose.

Steroid-sparing effect – Reducing the amount of steroid that is necessary to treat a particular condition.

Stratum corneum – The outermost layer of the outer layer (epidermis) of the skin. The cells of the stratum corneum are dead, but play an important role in protecting the body from the environment. The dead cells are continuously shed and replaced by new cells.

Streptococcus pyogenes – A bacterium from the *Streptococcus* family. Responsible for a variety of infections, including sore throat, scarlet fever, impetigo (small, pus-filled blisters on the skin), myositis (muscle inflammation) and acute inflammation of the kidneys.

Streptomyces tsukubaensis – A bacterium from the *Streptomyces* family, which live in soil and are similar in appearance to fungi. *Streptomyces* bacteria produce many compounds that are biologically active, including antibiotics. *Streptomyces tsukubaensis* produces the immunosuppressant drug tacrolimus, which is used in the treatment of atopic dermatitis.

Striae atrophicae – The medical term for stretch marks, bands of thin, wrinkled skin. The marks are initially red in appearance, but eventually turn purple and then white. Stretch marks commonly occur on the abdomen, buttock and thighs during puberty and pregnancy.

Subcapsular – Under the capsule or outer coating of the lens of the eye.

Superantigens – Toxins produced by certain bacteria and viruses that indiscriminately activate large numbers of T lymphocytes in the immune system, leading to inflammation throughout the body and other potentially fatal symptoms.

Surrogate markers – Laboratory or physical parameters that are used as a substitute for a direct biological measurement, such as how a patient feels or how effective a particular treatment is.

Symptom rebound – The recurrence of symptoms of a disease after suddenly stopping taking a drug for the treatment of that particular disease. The symptoms may be worse than they were before drug treatment was started.

Synthesis of proteins – The manufacture of proteins.

Systemic accumulation – The build-up of a substance in an organ or tissue.

Systemic – Pertaining to or affecting the entire body. Systemic treatment is treatment that reaches and affects cells throughout the body.

T-cell immunity – Also known as cellular immunity, T-cell immunity is the part of the body's immune response that results from the action of white blood cells known as T lymphocytes. See T lymphocytes.

T lymphocytes – A type of white blood cell found in blood and the lymphatic system. T lymphocytes play a major role in the body's immune response, and are activated by the presence of an antigen (invading organism). Following activation, they migrate to the site of the antigen where they either destroy the invading organism or activate other immune cells (e.g. macrophages and natural killer cells) to do so. There are a number of different types of T lymphocyte, including cytotoxic T cells, helper T cells, suppressor T cells and regulatory T cells.

Tachyphylaxis – A decrease in the response to a certain chemical (e.g. drug) following the continuous or repeated administration of the drug. That is to say, if a patient has been taking a drug for a few weeks, the beneficial effects of the drug may be less pronounced than they were at the start of treatment.

Telangiectasia – The permanent widening of small blood vessels in the skin, leading to a web-like pattern of small blood vessels on the surface of the skin.

Th1 cells – A subset of helper T lymphocytes which manufacture and secrete interleukin-2, γ-interferon and interleukin-12. Involved in the destruction of invading organisms.

Th2 cells – A subset of helper T lymphocytes which manufacture and secrete the interleukins (ILs), IL-4, IL-5, IL-6, and IL-10. Involved in humoral immunity, which is the production of antibodies by B lymphocytes.

Topical – On the surface of the body (i.e. the skin).

Topical steroids – A group of drugs that are applied to the surface of the skin for the treatment of skin conditions, including eczema and psoriasis. See Corticosteroids.

Topical triamcinolone acetonide – A corticosteroid that is applied to the surface of the skin for the treatment of inflammatory skin conditions, such as eczema and psoriasis. Also available as a nasal spray for the prevention and treatment of allergic rhinitis.

Transcriptional blockade – The blockade of transcription, the first step in the process of protein synthesis in cells.

Transcutaneous – Through the skin. A drug can be administered transcutaneously.

Transepidermal water loss – The loss of moisture through the epidermis (outer layer) of the skin.

Transforming growth factor (TGF)-β – A protein produced by a wide variety of tissues that acts as a signalling molecule. Has a paradoxical action, in that it can both stimulate and inhibit the growth of cells. Plays an important role in the biochemical pathways that help to keep the skin healthy.

Tryptase – An enzyme produced by activated mast cells that breaks down proteins. Plays a role in inflammatory allergic conditions, and is therefore a potential drug target for these conditions.

Tumour Necrosis Factor (TNF) – A cytokine that acts as a messenger between cells of the immune system. Produced by white blood cells in response to infection or the presence of cancer cells, and activates white blood cells to seek and destroy foreign substances (e.g. bacteria and viruses) and cancer cells. However, TNF also causes certain types of inflammation, such as that occurring in rheumatoid arthritis.

Tumour Necrosis Factor (TNF)-α – A member of the TNF family of cytokine proteins. TNF-α comprises 157 amino acids and has a wide range of proinflammatory actions. Two other types of TNF have been identified, β and γ. However, the term TNF (see previous entry) is often used synonymously with TNF-α.

Tumour necrosis factor (TNF)-β – A member of the TNF family of cytokine proteins. TNF-β, which is also known as lymphotoxin, shares many of the actions of TNF-α and is best known for its toxic effects on tumour cells.

Ultrasound examination – A technique used to produce an image of the inside of the body. High-frequency sound waves, which cannot be heard by the human ear, are passed into the body. The reflected echoes are picked up by a detector and analysed by a computer. The resulting image is then displayed on a television screen. Used to locate tumours within the body.

Undifferentiated lymphoma – A tumour of the lymphatic system (the tissues and organs in the body that carry a yellow fluid known as lymph and white blood cells that fight infection) that is composed of undifferentiated cells; cells that have not yet developed into any particular type of cell. Undifferentiated cancer cells often grow and spread quickly.

Up-regulation – An increase in the number of receptors for a certain chemical on the cell surface. This leads to an increase in the response that normally occurs when the relevant chemical binds to the receptor.

Urea – The waste product of protein metabolism in the body. Removed from the body in the urine via the kidneys.

UV-radiation phototherapy – Exposure to ultraviolet (UV) light for the treatment of certain skin conditions, such as vitiligo (white patches on the skin due to loss of pigment), eczema and psoriasis.

UV-free radiation – Artificial light that is free from ultraviolet (UV) rays.

Vaccination – The process of injecting a weakened or dead form of a disease (e.g. a virus) into patients to confer immunity against more serious forms of the disease. The weakened form of the disease stimulates the production of antibodies, which are then effective against the normal form of the disease, should the person contract it.

Varicose eczema – Eczema on the lower legs that is associated with the presence of varicose veins (swollen veins just under the skin). The affected skin is dry and itchy, and brown or purple patches may develop. Ultimately, ulcers may develop in the eczematous area.

Vascular cell adhesion molecule (VCAM)-1 – A glycoprotein (protein–sugar complex) present on the surface of endothelial cells (the cells lining the heart and blood vessels) that plays an important role in the immune response and inflammation. In particular, VCAM-1 helps to regulate the migration of immune cells into and out of the blood vessels.

Vehicle-controlled studies – Clinical trials in which the inactive ingredient of the treatment being tested (e.g. saline) is administered to some patients in order to show that the therapeutic effects of the drug are due to the active ingredient and not to the inactive ingredient.

Venipuncture – The piercing of a vein (usually in the forearm) with a hollow needle in order to withdraw blood or inject fluid.

Vesicles – Small, fluid-filled bumps (blisters) in the skin.

Useful contacts

The organisations listed below represent an accurate cross-section of what we believe to be reliable and up-to-date sources of information on eczema and its management.

British Association of Dermatologists

4 Fitzroy Square
London
W1T 5HQ
Email: *admin@bad.org.uk*
Tel: 0207 3830266
Website: *www.bad.org.uk*

The National Eczema Society

Highgate Hill
London
N19 5NA
Email: *helpline@eczema.org*
Helpline: 0870 241 3604
Website: *www.eczema.org*
Registered charity

Primary Care Dermatology Society

Gable House
40 High Street
Rickmansworth
Hertfordshire
WD3 1ER
Email: *pcds@pcds.org.uk*
Tel: 01923 711678
Website: *www.pcds.org.uk*
Registered charity

The Psoriasis Association

The Psoriasis Association
Milton House
7 Milton Street
Northampton
NN2 7JG
Email: *mail@psoriasis.demon.co.uk*
Tel: 0845 676 0076
Website: *www.psoriasis-association.org.uk*
Registered charity

The Skin Care Campaign

Website: *www.skincarecampaign.org*
Registered charity

Specialist Library: Skin Conditions

Website: *http://libraries.nelh.nhs.uk/skin*

Under My Skin

Website: *www.undermyskin.co.uk*

NHS Direct

Website: *www.nhsdirect.nhs.uk*

Best Treatments UK

Website: *www.besttreatments.co.uk*
Produced by the British Medical Association

British Dermatology Nurses Group

Website: *www.bdng.org.uk*

Index

Notes

Notes

Notes

Leading Healthcare Titles from CSF

BESTMEDICINE

www.bestmed.

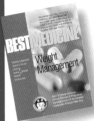

BESTMEDICINE
Weight Management
ISBN: 1-905064-91-8
£9.95, 240x190mm
128pp paperback
October 2004

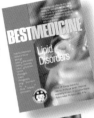

BESTMEDICINE
Lipid Disorders
ISBN: 1-905064-90-X
£12.95, 240x190mm
240pp paperback
October 2004

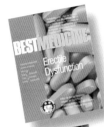

BESTMEL
Erectile D
ISBN: 1-905
£10.95, 24(
160pp pape
October 20(

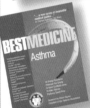

BESTMEDICINE
Asthma
ISBN: 1-905064-94-2
£13.95, 245x170mm
320pp paperback
April 2005

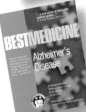

BESTMEDICINE
Alzheimer's Disease
ISBN: 1-905064-93-4
£12.95, 245x170mm
240pp paperback
April 2005

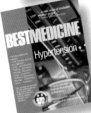

BESTMEL
Hyperten
ISBN: 1-905
£13.95, 24
320pp pape
April 2005

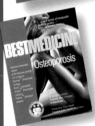

BESTMEDICINE
Osteoporosis
ISBN: 1-905064-81-0
£12.95, 245x170mm
240pp paperback
September 2005

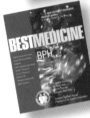

BESTMEDICINE
BPH
ISBN: 1-905064-96-9
£12.95, 245x170mm
240pp paperback
September 2005

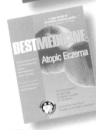

BESTMEL
Atopic Ec
ISBN: 1-905
£10.95, 245
160pp pape
September

OTHER TITLES: BESTMEDICINE COPD ISBN: 1-905064-97-7 October 2005
BESTMEDICINE Depression ISBN: 1-905064-98-5 February 2006
BESTMEDICINE Migraine ISBN: 1-905064-80-2 February 2006

PRIMARY CARE REVIEWS

www.csfme

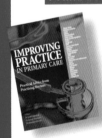

*Improving Practice
in Primary Care*
ISBN: 1-905064-82-9
£19.95, 240x190mm
336pp paperback
May 2005

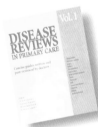

*Disease Reviews in
Primary Care Vol. 1*
ISBN: 1-905064-83-7
£17.95, 240x190mm
240pp paperback
May 2005

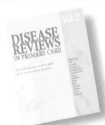

*Disease ▮
Primary (*
ISBN: 1-905
£17.95, 24(
240pp pape
May 2005

DRUGS IN CONTEXT

www.drugsinco.

The definitive
drug and
disease
management
resource

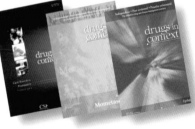

CSF Medical Communications Ltd, 1 Bankside, Lodge
Long Hanborough, Oxfordshire OX29 8LJ, UK
T: +44 (0)1993 885370 F: +44 (0)1993 88186
E: enquiries@csfmedical.com
CSF books are distributed by NBN International▮
Estover Road, Plymouth, PL7 7PY

Drugs in Context subscription details and back issues are available from
www.drugsincontext.com